KEYS TO HEALTH

_____

EDGAR CAYCE'S WISDOM FOR THE NEW AGE

General Editor: Charles Thomas Cayce
Project Editor: A. Robert Smith

KEYS TO HEALTH

The Promise and Challenge of Holism

ERIC A. MEIN, M.D.

With a Foreword by Charles Thomas Cayce

1817

Harper & Row, Publishers, San Francisco

New York, Grand Rapids, Philadelphia, St. Louis, London
Singapore, Sydney, Tokyo, Toronto

The author gratefully acknowledges the following publishers for permission to reprint from their publications:

Figure 2-1 (p. 22): Figure 2-16 from *Introduction to Psychology,* Sixth Edition, by Ernest R. Hilgard, Richard C. Atkinson, and Rita L. Atkinson, copyright © 1975 by Harcourt Brace Jovanovich, Inc., reprinted by permission of the publisher.

Figures 9-2 (p. 111) and **9-3** (p. 121): New Lifestyle Books for permission to reprint. © 1981 by Agatha Thrash, M.D. Used by permission

FIRST EDITION

Library of Congress Cataloging-in-Publication Data
Mein, Eric.
    Keys to health : the promise and challenge of holism / Eric Mein : with a foreword by Charles Thomas Cayce.—1st ed.
    p.   cm.
Bibliography: p.
Includes index.
ISBN 0-06-250594-7
    1. Holistic medicine.   2. Cayce, Edgar, 1877–1945.   3. Health.
4. Mental healing.   I. Title.
R733.M45   1989
613—dc20   89-45240
                                       CIP

ISBN 0-06-250594-7 (pbk.)

89 90 91 92 93 FAIR 10 9 8 7 6 5 4 3 2 1

To my parents,
John Gordon and Elizabeth,
for their love and support.

CONTENTS

FOREWORD

IT IS A TIME in the earth when people everywhere seek to know more of the mysteries of the mind, the soul," said my grandfather, Edgar Cayce, from an unconscious trance from which he demonstrated a remarkable gift for clairvoyance.

His words are prophetic even today, as more and more Americans in these unsettled times are turning to psychic explanations for daily events. For example, according to a national survey by the National Opinion Research Council nearly half of American adults today believe they have been in contact with someone who has died, a figure twice that of ten years ago. Two-thirds of all adults say they have had an ESP experience; ten years ago that figure was only one-half.

Every culture throughout history has made note of its own members' gifted powers beyond the five senses. These rare individuals held special interest because they seemed able to provide solutions to life's pressing problems. And America in the twentieth century is no exception.

Edgar Cayce was perhaps the most famous and most carefully documented psychic of our time. He began to use his unusual abilities when he was a young man, and from then on for over 40 years he would, usually twice a day, lie on a couch, go into a sleeplike state, and respond to questions. Over 14,000 of these discourses, called readings, were carefully transcribed by his secretary and preserved by the Edgar Cayce Foundation in Virginia Beach, Virginia. These psychic readings continue to provide inspiration, insight, and physical help to tens of thousands of people.

Having only an eighth-grade education, Edgar Cayce lived a plain and simple life by the world's standards. As early as his childhood in Hopkinsville, Kentucky, however, he sensed that he had psychic ability. While alone one day he had a vision of a woman who told him he would have unusual abilities to help people. He also related experiences of "seeing" dead relatives. Once, while struggling with school lessons, he slept on his spelling book and awakened knowing the entire contents of the book.

As a young man he experimented with hypnosis to treat a recurring throat problem that caused him to lose his speech. He discovered that under hypnosis he could diagnose and describe treatments for the physical ailments of others, often without knowing or seeing the person with the ailment. People began to ask him other sorts of questions and he found himself able to answer these as well.

In 1910 the *New York Times* published a two-page story with pictures about Edgar Cayce's psychic ability as described by a young physician, Wesley Ketchum, to a clinical research society in Boston. From that time on people from all over the country with every conceivable question sought his help.

In addition to his unusual talents, Cayce was a deeply religious man who taught Sunday school all of his adult life and read the entire Bible once for every year that he lived. He always tried to attune himself to God's will by studying the Scriptures and maintaining a rich prayer life, as well as by trying to be of service to those who came seeking help. He used his talents only for helpful purposes. Cayce's simplicity and humility and his commitment to doing good in the world continue to attract people to the story of his life and work and to the far-reaching information he gave.

In this series we hope to provide the reader with insights in the search for understanding and meaning in life. Each book in the series explores its subject from the viewpoint of the Edgar Cayce readings and compares the perspectives of other metaphysical literature and of current scientific thought. The interested reader needs no prior knowledge of the Edgar Cayce information. When one of the Edgar Cayce readings is quoted, the identifying number of that reading is included for those who may wish to read the full text. Each volume includes suggestions for further study.

This book, *Keys to Health: The Promise and Challenge of Holism*, by Eric A. Mein, M.D., is full of information to help you achieve an improved sense of well-being and prevent illness. Dr. Mein, who researched the book as a visiting scholar at the Edgar Cayce Foundation in Virginia Beach, Virginia, explains the common reasons for our becoming ill, and suggests ways of working with mental patterns to cope with stress and other debilitating conditions. He also outlines the Cayce treatments that proved successful in treating many diseases. Readers will find it a valuable addition to their home libraries for the most practical purpose—enjoying a healthy and fruitful life.

Charles Thomas Cayce, Ph.D.
President
Association for Research and Enlightenment

INTRODUCTION
AND ACKNOWLEDGMENTS

R ECENTLY, RESEARCHERS AT THE National Institutes of Health (NIH) began to examine whether a new approach to the treatment of cancer works. The technique involves removing some of the patient's blood, incubating it with Interleukin-2 (a molecule which is naturally present in our body and helps regulate the immune system), and then placing the mixture back in the patient. The hope is that the Interleukin-2 will stimulate the white blood cells that form the body's tumor surveillance system into heightened activity. The concept that the immune system might play a role in defending the body against cancer originated in the 1960s. It is still considered a novel idea and not universally accepted.

About 50 years ago, in 1940, Edgar Cayce gave a reading (no. 2208–1) for a 32-year-old doctor with acute myelogenous leukemia, a virulent malignancy of the bone marrow. In this reading, Cayce suggests taking this individual's blood, mixing it with a small quantity of tincture of iodine to "activate" the cells, and placing it back in the body with the next transfusion. Unfortunately, the young doctor died 5 days after the reading was given and before anyone had a chance to work with the idea given in his reading. The readings are clear that this concept is experimental and would require refinement.

They make similar suggestions to "culture" the blood of several other individuals with cancer as well.

In other readings, given in the 1920s, 1930s, and 1940s, Cayce clearly speaks of cancer being able to take hold because of the "low vitality in the system of the leukocyte [the immune system]." Many of the recommended cancer therapies were intended to "prepare the blood stream against the tentacles of the condition from going deeper. . . ."

Remarkable? This is but one example of the information in the Cayce physical readings that struck me during the year I spent examining them as a "scholar-in-residence" at Atlantic University. Of the 14,145 transcribed readings, *68 percent* are classified as "physical readings"—dealing directly with the physical complaints and conditions of individuals who came to Cayce for his help. As I studied these, I arrived at the following conclusions:

- There is a remarkable consistency throughout the physical readings. They present a deep, beautiful, and coherent picture of how the body functions in health and disease. This fact emerges when *all* the readings on a given topic are examined at the same time, as they are in Part Two of this book. When analyzed in this fashion, they contain insights from which generalizations can be drawn.

- The therapies prescribed by the readings *do not* rely heavily on magical or "vibratory influences" which science will never understand. Unlike most "holistic therapies," the readings not only begin with spiritual premises, they also are equally at home in the world of the cell, agreeing with science that the pathology of disease occurs at this level and that therapies need to be directed here. From the readings' perspective, the body lives in the world of cause-and-effect. All of the recommended therapies have very real effects on the body which can be documented—from castor oil acting as a prostaglandin precursor to adjustments working with facilitated neurons. If that sounds complex, it should. That's the point! While the readings couch these concepts in the language of a poet/mystic, they are

scientific and are interpretable and testable. The physical readings themselves invite this scrutiny.

- Despite the advances that science has made during the past 50
  years, the concepts in the readings are still worth further exploration. In many ways, medicine is slowly catching up with the
  readings. We now rely heavily on a drop of blood for diagnosis.
  The essentials of the "Cayce diet" agree completely with those
  now suggested by the American Cancer Society and the American Heart Association. As noted above, the concept that the
  immune system protects the body from cancer was first proposed in the 1960s—the readings clearly discussed it in the
  1920s, 1930s, and 1940s. There are still many ideas in the
  readings which are very innovative. Some of these, like the importance of nerve reflexes in asthma, are just one step beyond
  what science knows. Others, like the role of gold in multiple
  sclerosis, or the importance of the potassium/iodine balance in
  thyroid disorders, or the place of colonics in the treatment of
  coronary heart disease, are completely new and exciting ideas.
  Furthermore, the readings, in their approach to healing, present a coherent philosophy which is fundamentally different
  from the current medical approach and deserves examination.

- The bottom line on the readings' accuracy and applicability is
  still not known. They have never been worked with in a systematic manner or had their efficacy closely scrutinized. There
  are many anecdotal stories of success. There are also some bla-
  tant errors. The readings themselves are not magical, not now
  or when they were first given. Every single suggestion demanded effort—physical, mental, and spiritual—on the part
  of the patient and those working with the patient. Each recommended therapy, while given to an individual, was based on
  a given set of principles which should still be valid 44 years
  after Edgar Cayce's death. The final word on whether the
  Cayce approach to health is the right one awaits the testing of
  these concepts.

I have written this book with three purposes in mind. The first is to explain the basic principles contained in the Edgar Cayce readings of how the body functions in health and disease. I have tried to do this in a manner which makes the principles understandable while also trying to be complete and true to the readings' approach. The second purpose is to provide the reader with enough practical information to apply these principles. Finally, I have written this book in the hope that it will help stimulate enough interest and excitement about this information to generate the needed research to test these concepts and get them into the mainstream. To help promote this research, I have founded Meridian Institute. If you would like more information about this effort, please contact me at the address provided in the author information section at the rear of this book.

I am grateful to Atlantic University and the Edgar Cayce Foundation for sponsoring my year of exploration of the readings. I would also like to thank Herb Puryear for early discussions which first led to my fascination with the material in the readings. Thanks also go to Mae St. Clair for sharing her knowledge accumulated from working with the readings for the past 50 years. Joseph Dunn has ably served as my editor and I am grateful for his help. Finally, and most importantly, I am deeply thankful to my wife, Cathy, and my children, Rachael and Christopher, for giving my life meaning and balance and for their patience during this project.

PART I

The Cayce Paradigm

1

The Promise and the Challenge: The Central Premise

Thy body is the temple that must be, should be, will *be kept holy, if ye will know thy true relationships to thy Maker.*
EDGAR CAYCE reading no. 261–15*

The real voyage of discovery consists not in seeking new lands but in seeing with new eyes.
MARCEL PROUST

In 1977 THE MEDIA reported the moving story of a boy named David, who had lived all his life inside a plastic bubble in a Houston, Texas, hospital. The air he breathed in this specially controlled, germ-free environment was filtered to remove any bacteria, viruses, or other foreign substances. His food was sterilized and

---

*Each of the Edgar Cayce readings has been assigned a two-part number to provide easy reference. Each person who received a reading was given an anonymous number; this is the first half of the two-part number. Since many individuals obtained more than one reading, the second number designates the number of that reading in the series. Reading no. 261–15 was given for a person who was assigned case number 261. This particular reading was the fifteenth one this person obtained from Cayce.

served through airlocks. Because his immune system was nonfunctional, David was required to live a life of complete isolation. At age twelve, he was removed from his bubble for a bone-marrow transplant in an attempt to give him his freedom. For the first time, David was able to feel his mother's kiss. Sadly, the transplant was unsuccessful and David died of complications from the operation. He had, however, lived longer than any human being without a functioning immune system.

A story like David's heightens our awareness of how much we take our bodies for granted. You and I do not need to live in a bubble, isolated from the world. Yet, each day we come in contact with viruses and bacteria by the millions. In fact, there are numerous potential pathogens on the pages you are reading. Despite such encounters, we go through our daily routines unperturbed by these microscopic attackers, relying on our body's wisdom to sometimes resist, sometimes tolerate, and sometimes actually encourage their growth. Infections occur only when there is a breakdown in the constant negotiations between host and visitor, resulting in one side overstepping its borders. This occurrence, however, is the exception rather than the rule.

This amazing capacity to balance on the tightrope of health extends beyond our immune systems. Whether walking on the beach on a warm August day or on a cold January morning, our body's temperature is maintained at 98.6° F. Similarly, almost regardless of what we eat, our blood makeup stays constant. It is this inner wisdom that allows us to recover from illnesses and other assaults on our well-being.

A simple example of this innate healing ability that we often take for granted is wound repair. The entire sequence of events—from the wound bleeding to cleanse itself to the blood clotting to form a scab to the redness and warmth signaling that the white blood cells have arrived to remove the debris and defend against infection—is a thing of beauty. This process has been so perfected that healing usually occurs without loss of sensation or movement in the area of the cut.

Most doctors recognize the body's ability to heal itself; certainly all depend on it. The old cliché, "Take two aspirin and call me in the morning," reflects the knowledge that the body, given time, can re-store itself. Doctors, however, usually don't advertise this secret.

Norman Cousins tells the story of having asked Dr. Albert Schweitzer to explain the success of witch-doctor healers. Schweitzer responded that Cousins was asking him to divulge a secret that doctors had carried ever since Hippocrates. Dr. Schweitzer continued, "The witch doctor succeeds for the same reason all the rest of us succeed. Each patient carries his own doctor inside him. They come to us not knowing this truth. We are at our best when we give the doctor who resides within each patient a chance to go to work."

Put more succinctly and less romantically over 200 years ago by Voltaire, "The art of medicine consists of amusing the patient while nature cures the disease." Far from being a passive victim to disease, the human body can rally its healing forces and remove the offender or repair damaged tissue with more vigor than the world's best-trained medical team.

How does the body do this? What is the source of this healing? Science acknowledges that it doesn't know the answers to these questions; that they constitute a true mystery. The Cayce readings, however, are clear in the answers they give to these questions—and the answers form the principle on which *all* the information in the Cayce health readings is based.

The Cayce readings strongly emphasize that the body's innate healing ability is the direct result of the manifestation of Spirit within it. "For, all healing must come from the Divine. . . . The Source of the Universal supply" (no. 4021–1). Over and over again, the readings drive home the point that healing can come from only one source—God.

Healing requires the "attuning [of] each atom . . . to the aware-ness of the divine that lies within each atom, each cell of the body" (no. 3384–2). "And whether there is the applicaton of foods, exer-cise, medicine, or even the knife, it is to bring the consciousness . . . of creative or God forces" (no. 2696–1).

Amazing! These last three quotes from the readings—examples of many similar ones—form the core of a coherent and deep philos-ophy of healing.

True healing *requires* an inner response. When Jesus said, "Thy faith has made thee whole" (Matthew 9:22), he was directly acknowledging a physical transformation caused by the Spirit within. When this Spirit was absent, even Jesus could not help the blind to see and the lame to walk.

Medicine regularly encounters the body's inner healing ability whenever it attempts to study the body. Researchers, in fact, find it almost impossible to escape from it and consider it a nuisance. Because of this, it is often assigned a negative connotation and given a derogatory name: the placebo response. The lowly placebo response, however, provides dramatic proof of the body's innate healing potentials.

One example of the body's power is its success in dealing with the mundane wart. There is extensive evidence that warts are often best dealt with by suggestion alone. Nonsensical remedies and plain hypnotic suggestion will cause warts to disappear. Physician-author Lewis Thomas wrote that "this is . . . more of a surprise than cloning, recombinant DNA or endorphins or acupuncture or anything else currently attracting the press. . . . It illustrates there has to be a Person in charge, running matters of meticulous detail beyond anyone's comprehension, a skilled engineer and manager, a chief executive—and a world class cell biologist."

A more dramatic example of the placebo response can be found in two studies done in the late 1950s. Completed before there were committees to oversee the ethics of experimentation, both studies compared the effects of "sham surgery," in which the patient is cut open and then closed with nothing else done, to internal mammary artery ligation, the operation of choice at that time for the treatment of angina pectoris. The two studies had similar results. Both groups showed improvement of their symptoms, with the "sham surgery" group actually doing slightly better than those who had the full surgical procedure.

The implications of such examples are often ignored by physicians. As you can imagine, a placebo response can be embarassing to a clinician. It implies a patient got better in spite of, not because of, the therapy given. The body's healing ability is recognized as the reason many healing methods used in the past gave the illusion of being effective. As many scholars point out, the history of medicine is also the history of the placebo response. Most current-day physicians want to separate themselves as far as possible from this history and the days of "nonscientific medicine."

The point that such doctors miss is that a placebo response is evidence that a patient's consciousness has been impacted by the therapy given, facilitating actual healing by the doctor within. This healing is as real as if a pill had changed the body's physiology. From the perspective of the Cayce readings, the placebo response is to be welcomed and even sought, not avoided.

This healing ability is, in fact, the evidence that we are spiritual beings. The Cayce readings propose that spiritual forces manifest in our world as the "reproductive principle." Our cells' ability to renew or regenerate themselves is the most fundamental of universal laws and, according to the readings, is the first principle of spiritual forces.

Such a principle makes even more sense when we look around us and see that healing is a universal property of all of creation. Life everywhere naturally tends toward wholeness and growth. Animals and plants are able to heal themselves without the help of a doctor. Whole ecosystems heal themselves. Take, for example, a field in which the trees have been cut. It will go through a slow process of regeneration—first with grasses, then with brush, and finally the return of trees. Even stars are capable of healing themselves as evidenced by Nova explosions.

The Cayce readings indicate that the ability to renew and reproduce ourselves is evidence of a promise from God. Our bodies contain within them the pattern to be whole and are continuously trying to achieve that pattern. To accomplish this, "Each and every atomic structure of the body is able to reproduce itself, and is continually doing so; from the tiniest cell to the functioning of the larger organs . . ." (no. 1158–11).

That seems straightforward. We have all experienced our body's healing ability. However, when one thinks through the concept that such healing is the spiritual heritage of each of our cells, there are some dramatic implications:

- First, if there is a pattern within every cell for its proper functioning, how do we become ill? The simple healing philosophy just presented leads to some startling conclusions about the origin and meaning of illness, which will be explored in Chapter Three.

- Second, the Latin phrase *primum non noceri* (first do no harm), which is part of the oath every physician takes on graduation, takes on an entirely new meaning. The prime directive for all healers and practitioners would be: "above all, do not impede the body's own healing ability." Our approach to the body should be one of awe and a desire to assist it rather than one of arrogance. With such an approach, the large number of tonsillectomies and the radiation of children's thymus glands would not have occurred and the present rash of appendectomies, hysterectomies, and injudicious use of medications would be gone.

- Third, no single therapeutic approach to the body holds all the answers. Since all healing comes from within, it follows that "Not by the methods does the healing come, though the consciousness of the individual is such that this or that method is the one that is more effective in the individual case" (no. 969–1). In other words, for a similar sore throat, one person may respond best to penicillin while another may respond more quickly to a castor oil pack applied over the area. All systems, in fact, demonstrate both cures and failures. Despite great inconsistencies in their methods, they all seem to work at times.

- Fourth, the best therapeutic systems are those which work with, not against, the body's own healing abilities. The readings explain this is why they recommend osteopathy and hydrotherapy more frequently than any other treatments.

- Fifth, suppression of symptoms should not be confused with healing. Quieting the cells with a medicinal curfew may at times give the illusion of success, but may make matters worse.

- Sixth, we should be able to help almost any condition. The Cayce readings constantly remind those seeking advice that the body gradually and constantly renews itself. Hence, one's present state of health is always to be viewed as something which can be built on and improved. One individual asked if it was possible to help those with incurable diseases. Cayce, in reading no. 3744–1, replied, "There are in truth no incurable conditions, that which is was produced from some force." This reading went on to say that any force could be counteracted and a given situation improved.

- Seventh, prevention of and cure of a condition often require the same steps. Both require working with and changing the pattern creating the problem. An example is the disease process of atherosclerosis, the buildup of plaques in our arteries which can lead to heart attacks and strokes. Science and the readings tell us that if we take the cells that line our arteries, put them in an environment filled with fat or cholesterol, and increase the pressure of the blood around them, they will start to form plaques. Obviously, if we want to prevent the plaques from forming, we should alter our diet to lower our cholesterol and make sure our blood pressure stays within the normal range. However, if the promise of renewal as found in the readings is true, we should be able to change the environment around the cells forming one of these plaques and see the cells change their pattern from one of destruction to one of healing. This is, in fact, the case. Recent studies have shown that when individuals decrease their cholesterol, and this is only a single factor causing the problem, 80 percent or more of them will see no further progression in the size of their plaques or will get an actual reduction in the plaques' size.

So what appears to be a simple premise—the body contains the wisdom or the pattern to heal itself and will do so when given the chance—has major ramifications. Every therapy used in the Cayce readings emerges from, and is consistent with, this premise. The primary objective of these therapies is to work with the body's own healing ability, coordinating each system to work in harmony with the whole. These therapies aim for a gentle improvement of the whole body, never the pitting of one force against another to merely suppress symptoms.

This approach is in stark contrast to the way medicine is practiced today in the U.S., where war and battle imagery dominate the thinking. Researchers are continually looking for new "magic bullets" to add to doctors' "therapeutic arsenals." As a society, we demand that scientists find "new weapons to win the war against disease." Dr. Andrew Weil, in his book *Health and Healing: Understanding Conventional and Alternative Medicine*, concludes that the result of all this is that "the body of the average allopathic* patient becomes a perpetual war zone for the testing and use of therapeutic weaponry [and] the best hope is for an occasional cease-fire."

We also can see the effect of this battle-oriented mentality in the nation's prescription patterns. The three most prescribed drugs in 1983 were Cimetidine, Inderal, and Valium. Cimetidine blocks the stomach's secretion of acid. Inderal blocks the sympathetic nervous system in order to control blood pressure and anxiety. Valium blocks our moods. As a nation, we swallow 25 million pills every hour; many of them to block the symptoms of underlying processes we have little understanding of. So, despite the 200 years since his observation, Voltaire's words still ring true today: "Physicians pour drugs of which they know little, to cure diseases of which they know less, into humans of which they know nothing."

Before being accused of tearing apart allopathy, which *has* had some spectacular successes, there is a need to acknowledge that, as individuals and as a society, *we* have demanded the "magic bullet." *We* have placed medicine under constant pressure to provide explanations for the causes of diseases and to provide immediate cures. *We* are the ones who go to the doctor expecting instant relief and the

---

*Allopathy— term coined by Samuel Hahnemann, father of homeopathy, to describe the use of remedies that produce effects different from the symptoms of the disease. The term is now used to describe traditional Western medicine as practiced by most medical doctors in the United States.

prerequisite prescription before we are willing to leave the office. We are, in effect, asking doctors to be responsible for our health.

One reason for this is that most of us take our bodies for granted and know very little about them. We usually know more about our cars than our bodies and we tend to take better care of the auto. If a study came out tomorrow showing that smoking cigarettes in a car instantly corroded the engine, smokers would quit smoking in their car. Similarly, many people pay more for premium gas to get better performance from their engine. Yet their next stop will be at a greasy-food restaurant where they will put anything into their own system. Likewise, most people regularly change the oil and get tune-ups for their cars, but rarely take the time to tune up their own bodies.

In some ways, our bodies are like cars. Both will run when their valves are burnt, when they are passing oil and leaking noxious exhaust fumes, when their brakes are worn, and when their steering is loose. Both can be taken to the best mechanics in town to have them fixed after they break down. However, mechanics can't prevent us from abusing either our bodies or our cars and causing future problems. Unlike our cars, our bodies can't be traded in. Preventive maintenance and care in driving *and* in living will save a great deal of expense and effort.

While there are no Cayce readings equating our bodies to automobiles, the readings make comparisons which indicate we should hold the workings of our body in awe:

> There is no greater factory in the universe than that in a human body in its natural, normal reacting state (no. 1800–21).

> The human anatomical body is as the working of a perfect whole of a piece of machinery, and that—kept in the proper working order—will perform the function of not only furnishing its own fuel for operation but supply that necessary for replenishing that fuel. (no. 4999–1)

As science explores the body, it adds details that reinforce this sense of wonder. For example, the heart beats a hundred thousand times every 24 hours and pumps 6,300 gallons of blood a day through 96,000 miles of blood vessels. To replenish this blood, 3 million new red blood cells are created every second. When one realizes that these are only a few of the thousands of operations continually going on in our body, one has to be filled with a sense of awe. The fact that our 70 trillion cells, each containing ten thousand more molecules than the Milky Way has stars, work in a coordinated fashion is, indeed, a miracle.

Fully able to perceive this miracle, the Cayce readings repeatedly used the biblical analogy that our "body is the temple of the Holy Spirit" (1 Corinthians 6:19). The readings carry the analogy further by stating that our body serves as a temple for our soul, that God will meet us within this temple, and, thus, we can find the kingdom of heaven inside ourselves. But the readings also repeatedly say that this will be a difficult, if not impossible, task unless we set that temple in order.

So, with the promise of renewal comes the challenge of having total responsibility for shaping our bodies. The New Testament tells the story of Jesus going into the temple in Jerusalem, finding it corrupted, and throwing out the moneychangers, asking them, "What have you done to my Father's house?" The following reading reflects a similar frankness:

> And when there are rebellions of body or mind against such, is there any wonder that the atoms of the body cause high blood pressure, or cause itching, or cause running sores, or cause a rash, or cause indigestion? For, all of these are but the rebellion of truth and light, error and correction in a physical body.
>
> For thy body is indeed the Temple of the Living God. What have you dragged into this Temple? (no. 3174–1)

Like a temple, the body needs to "be kept purified [and] cleansed; as you would for *any* service to that ye would worship!" (no. 2067–3).

Each of us needs to take stock of how well we are keeping our temple. Take a few minutes now to complete the Health Inventory in Figure 1-1. There are no trick questions to test your honesty and you will find it easy to tell the most desirable answer. As a result, your score reflects your concept of your state of well-being. More important than the score is what you learn about yourself in the process.

Figure 1-1:   My health inventory

No or never	Rarely	Some-times	Often	Yes or usually	
0	1	2	3	4	
——	——	——	——	——	1. I sleep well.
——	——	——	——	——	2. I am fairly steady in my moods.
——	——	——	——	——	3. I have a good appetite.
——	——	——	——	——	4. I have three colds a year or less.
——	——	——	——	——	5. Unless I'm working hard or the weather is hot my hands do not perspire.
——	——	——	——	——	6. I have a bowel movement at least once a day.
——	——	——	——	——	7. It is easy for me to stay alert and concentrate.
——	——	——	——	——	8. I am within 15 pounds of my ideal weight.
——	——	——	——	——	9. I have good feelings about my body.
——	——	——	——	——	10. My respirations are deep and regular.
——	——	——	——	——	11. When I sit, I am relaxed and my spine is relatively straight.
——	——	——	——	——	12. I am free of aches and pains.
——	——	——	——	——	13. My skin is clear, without acne or rashes.
——	——	——	——	——	14. I feel energetic and have good stamina.
——	——	——	——	——	15. I can touch my toes easily with my hands when standing with knees straight.
——	——	——	——	——	16. My hands and feet generally stay warm.
——	——	——	——	——	17. I am happy in my personal relationships.
——	——	——	——	——	18. I have a sense of well being.
——	——	——	——	——	19. I am free of headaches.
——	——	——	——	——	20. I do something for fun at least once a week.
——	——	——	——	——	21. I do not abuse drugs or alcohol.
——	——	——	——	——	22. I do not depend on medicines, including prescription drugs, to maintain my health.
——	——	——	——	——	23. When I awaken in the morning, I am not overly stiff.
——	——	——	——	——	24. Silence is enjoyable.
——	——	——	——	——	25. I have a personal definition of God which has meaning to me.

————Total Score

Scoring: 75–100—Fantastic! Remember, an ounce of prevention . . .

       50–75—Join the crowd, we all could be better.

       25–50—Time to get cracking.

Less than 25—If you are not already under the care of a health professional, please go see one immediately.

If you didn't score 100, don't despair. All of us have room for improvement in our health and all of us are given lots of time for that improvement. One person asked if he could perfect the body. The reading responded that it was possible, but it would take this individual a minimum of thirty lifetimes. If that's overwhelming, the readings also tell us that nothing is asked of any soul except to do what we know to do today. As we apply what we know day by day, the next step will be given.

Lao-Tsu, author of the *Tao Te Ching*, tells us that "the journey of a thousand miles begins with one step." Similarly, the Cayce readings advise us to begin where we are. Each of us knows better than anyone else "that which has hindered them from being physically, mentally, and spiritually in accord with the divine that *is* life manifested in the body" (no. 294–202). If we take just a moment to look inside ourselves, we already know of something that we should eliminate and something we need to encourage in our lifestyle. Before you continue this book in search of new ideas, it is important to begin working with what you already know. Take a moment now to think of several of these. Then, make a choice for change today.

I will eliminate _____

_____

_____

_____

I will encourage _____

_____

_____

_____

For the next 7 days work consistently at making these changes in your life.

Philosophers through the ages have recognized the importance and the challenge of the admonition "know thyself." They and the

Cayce readings agree that such a lesson is our ultimate study. As we become more familiar with our inner healing systems, we will be able to use the skills of the doctor within, just as we are able to use our skills of reading, writing, or driving a car. As we are able to do that, we will be transformed from the role of a passive victim when we are ill to the role of an active and skillful healer of our own bodies.

An ancient Greek thinker once said, "Give me a place to stand on and I will move the earth." The rest of this book will attempt to give you such a place to stand on.

2

The Body Triune: Spiritual, Mental, and Physical

It is highly dishonorable for a reasonable soul to live in so divinely built a mansion as the body she resides in altogether unacquianted with the exquisite structure of it.
ROBERT BOYLE

The love of and for a pure body is the most sacred experience in an entity's earthly sojourn.
EDGAR CAYCE reading no. 436–2

IN 1978, A BABY girl was conceived in a petri dish. This first "test-tube baby" shocked and amazed the world. More mysterious, however, is the much older miracle—how a solitary sperm can join with an egg and become a human being. No one has the foggiest notion of how the original cell moves through time and space to become the 70 trillion cells which eventually will write poems, play soccer, or devise new inventions. This is one of the *ultimate* questions. One medical philosopher has promised to have skywriting planes fill the sky with exclamation points if someone ever provides the answer.

If we are to accept the challenge of caring for our bodies as a sacred heritage, we need to understand our bodies as best we can. The Cayce readings propose that our formation is both far from haphazard and is filled with symbology. ". . . the physical body is a pattern of the universal consciousness" (no. 2787–1). One physician was told in a reading to study the Book of the Revelation side-by-side with an anatomy atlas to better understand the body. Elsewhere, the readings compare the stages of fetal development to the Old Testament account of Jewish history. While these esoteric descriptions of the body are fascinating, they are also difficult to interpret. The readings, however, also contain many easily understood concepts which can help us on our prilgrimage to health.

A first generalization is that the microcosm reflects the macrocosm. This is a useful concept in several ways. First, the readings tell us that we can best understand our bodies as being composed of three parts, symbolically reflecting the three-dimensional world in which we live. There is a physical body, a mental body, and a spiritual body. Each is a separate part of us and, at the same time, they are one and the same thing. An analogy might be made to a corn plant which is composed of many parts, including leaves, stalk, and roots. There is also the ear of corn which, like the physical body, bears the fruit of the whole. While all these components form the one corn plant, their functions are distinct and different.

The Cayce readings also compare the relationship of these three bodies to the Christian mystery of the Trinity—Father, Son, and Holy Ghost. Three in one. Separate and yet the same thing. Each needing to be worked within its own realm and yet one constantly affecting the others.

Scientists are recognizing that no line can be drawn between psyche and soma, mind and body. Continuums of staggering complexity involving sophisticated communication systems are becoming evident. Researchers in such fields as psychoneuroimmunology—which looks at the interaction of our thoughts, immune systems, and nervous systems—have begun to speak of an integrated "bodymind." Every system of the body they have thus far examined—the autonomic nervous system, the glands of the endocrine system, the brain's neurotransmitters, and the immune system—has been implicated as participating in this dialogue, leading one well-known researcher to proclaim that, "Clearly, the conceptual division between the sciences of immunology, endocrinology, and psychology/neuroscience is a historical artifact."

A premise in the Cayce readings which helps us to understand the functions, separately and together, of each of the three bodies is the Spirit is the life, Mind is the builder, and the Physical is the result.

THE SPIRIT IS THE LIFE

Spirit is the reproductive principle and, as the essence of life, can be accessed equally by all—be it the brainy individual or the babe. The readings indicate that the spiritual body is not contained within the physical. But "there is the pattern in the material or physical plane of every condition as exists in the cosmic or spiritual plane . . ." (no. 5756–4).

The physical points of contact for our spiritual bodies are our glands, which "secrete that which enables the body, physically throughout, to *reproduce* itself!" (no. 1475–1).

Glands release small amounts of very potent molecules which strongly influence the body. The pituitary, for example, secretes at least ten hormones but weighs only one-fiftieth of an ounce. Its daily output of these substances is only one-millionth of a gram. This, however, is enough to regulate the thyroid, adrenals, gonads, and our growth. One of these hormones is so powerful that it can be detected by biological assay in a dilution of one part in 15 billion. To obtain that dilution, one ounce of hormone can be mixed with the water contained in 418,080 tanker trucks, each holding two thousand gallons of water. Powerful stuff!

These glands also help determine our character and disposition. Their physiology often reflects our approach in spirit to our purpose or motivation. While the capacity for regeneration pertains to all the body's glands, the readings identify seven glands as playing an especially important role as the seven major spiritual centers of our body, equivalent to Hinduism's chakras. These vortexes of energy are identified by the readings as the gonads, the cells of Leydig, the adrenals, the thymus, the thyroid, the pineal, and the pituitary. As transmitters of energy, these seven centers play an important role in our connection with the Divine.

Our health begins in the spiritual realm; however, the physical manifestations of ill health rarely affect the glands. The most common of the seven glands to be affected by illness are the thyroid and the adrenals. These two have the most neuronal contact with the autonomic nervous system and the readings suggest that is why they run into problems more often than the others.

The major reason to direct therapy at the glands, based on the readings, is the role they play in helping each cell and organ reproduce. The use of small cyclic doses of Atomidine is the most frequent method given by the readings to help the glands function. Atomidine is a form of iodine which apparently is helpful and not toxic to the body when correctly used. Occasionally, iodine and gold used with the wet-cell appliance are suggested to enhance glandular functioning as well (see Chapter Ten).

MIND IS THE BUILDER

If all of us are gifted with the same Spirit, what sets us apart as individuals? The answer, according to the Cayce readings, is the patterns within our mental bodies. The analogy of a film projector can help us understand this concept. The light bulb and projected light represent the Spirit. The images on the screen are the result—the physical manifestation. The film, which patterns the light to create the images, is comparable to our mental body. It is here that the patterns leading to health or illness are created.

Where is the home of these patterns? Is it the brain? We know we can affect the conscious mind with medicines and drugs. Metabolic disorders as simple as low or high blood sugar will also affect the ability of our mind to work. Neurosurgeons can stimulate areas of the brain and produce movements, sensations, emotions, and bring back memories. With such evidence, one might assume that our brain is our mind. The readings say no: "Thy *brain* is not thy mind, it is that which is used by thy mind!" (no. 826–11) When one turns the tuning knob on their television set, the picture becomes distorted. Likewise, the fact that a drug like LSD can distort our perceptions doesn't automatically imply our minds do not reach beyond the physical.

The position taken by the readings is that our mental bodies are half in the physical and half removed from it. If we are spiritual beings, this makes sense. To retain an awareness when we die, part of our mind must be separate from the physical apparatus which houses it in this dimension.

The Cayce material holds this position in excellent company. William Penfield, the neurosurgeon who first mapped the brain, wrote in his last book, *The Mystery of the Mind*, that all of the mind is not coextensive with the brain. Nobel laureate John Eccles agrees, contending that the brain is but the receiver—like a radio or television set—for the signals sent by a mind that is separate from it.

This concept is also supported by the well-known research of Karl Lashley in the 1930s. Lashley went in search of memory and was unable to localize it. No one portion of the brain could be removed to destroy a particular memory. Likewise, the more brain removed, no matter which part, the dimmer the memory became. Lashley concluded that memory was contained in the entire brain.

From other experiments, we have learned that the mind will adapt to the receiving set—the brain. When volunteers put on contact lenses that literally turned their world upside down, the mind, in only a few days, adapted and perceived the world right side up again.

There are cases in the scientific literature of individuals who have had an entire hemisphere, or half, of their brain removed to help with untreatable epilepsy and who have retained normal language and intellectual abilities. Similarly, in 1980, British neurologist John Lorber published observations on people with hydrocephaly—a condition in which the normal fluid-filled spaces in the head have enlarged, compressing the brain tissue. He cited one young student in particular "who has an IQ of 126, has gained a first-class honors degree in mathematics, and is socially completely normal. And yet the boy has virtually no brain." Instead of the normal 45-millimeter thickness of outer cortex, a CAT scan found just a "thin layer of mantle measuring a millimeter or so."

The Cayce readings divide our nervous system into three components: the cerebrospinal system consisting of the brain and spinal cord, the sympathetic nervous system (part of our autonomic nervous system which usually operates outside our voluntary control), and the sensory nervous system. The coordination of these three is vital to our well-being. Of these, the significance of the sympathetic nervous system is the most underestimated. This system communicates directly with each of our organs and glands, innervates and controls each of our blood vessels, and helps regulate our immune systems. It is composed of two chains of nerves that run along either side of our spinal cord.

The readings state that it is the sympathetic nervous system which is "the brain manifestation of soul forces in the body" (no. 4566–1). When asked what is the control center of our mental bodies, the readings named the solar plexus—a large gathering of nerves in our upper abdomen which is part of the sympathetic nervous system.

It is in our autonomic nervous system that our subconscious—90 percent of our awareness—resides. Any attempts at healing need to take this into account. Otherwise, like an iceberg, if only the surface material is chipped away, more of the same will rise above the water to take its place.

THE PHYSICAL IS THE RESULT

Our bodies are the direct results of our thoughts (the patterns we've created) and the building blocks we've brought into them (through what we've eaten). They also directly reflect the concept of "as the macrocosm, so the microcosm." Like the earth, our bodies are three-quarters water, and the blood running through us is essentially seawater in its composition.

This relationship is repeated again at the level of the cell, once again reflecting the macrocosm: ". . . every cell of the body is a universe in itself . . ." (no. 1158–22). Each of the 70 trillion cells in our

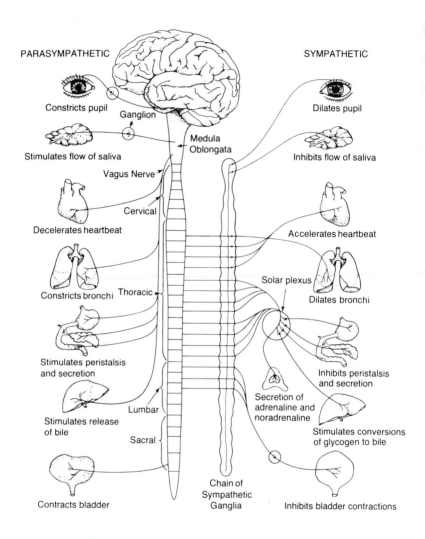

Figure 2-1. The autonomic nervous system.

bodies is too small to be seen without a microscope. But each is still about 1 billion times the size of their smallest components. Like us, each cell is a droplet of seawater contained by a membrane, consisting of thousands of working parts. Like us, they contain power stations, a transportation system, and an elaborate communications setup. And like us, there is no such thing as "the typical cell." They come in a variety of shapes and with a myriad of functions.

Despite their diversity, each cell contains the whole. Within each are the blueprints to create an entire baby. If you took all the DNA from your 70 trillion cells it would fit into a box the size of an ice cube. But if you unwound it—the string would stretch to the sun and back four hundred times.

The Cayce readings emphasize that each of these 70 trillion cells has it own awareness. Often in our arrogance, we assume that our day-to-day consciousness, based in the outermost layer of cells—only 0.1 inches thick—of our cortex, is the totality of our awareness. We forget that this contains only a small fraction of our 10 billion neurons.

A fascinating perspective on this has emerged from recent testing of individuals who have had the 200 million fibers connecting the two halves of their brains—the corpus callosum—cut as a treatment for severe epilepsy. Each hemisphere in these individuals completely controls the opposite side of the body and receives sensory input from only the left or the right visual field. The word "heart" was flashed in front of these individuals in such a way that the right side of the brain saw "he" and the left saw "art" (he/art). When asked what word they had seen, the left cortex, which usually controls the speech center, would answer "art." When asked to point at the word with their left hand (controlled by the right side of the brain), they would point at the word "he," often while verbally stating "no, that's not right" and showing embarrassment.

Each side of the brain had an awareness that the other side had no idea existed. It is equally possible that there are areas and levels of awareness in our own bodies of which our thin cortexes know little about.

Hans Selye, a well-known physiologist, found that single cells "can respond with many more or less specific, qualitatively different biologic reaction forms." In other words, they respond with an awareness of their environment. This includes adapting to different situations and even changing from one type of a cell to another.

Lymphocytes, a type of cell in our immune systems, are classic examples of this. They spend their lives in exploration through the body, sensing and monitoring, often pushing upstream through the blood in search of foreign invaders. Once found, the lymphocytes proceed through an elaborate interaction with each other, leading to action and the creation of memory within these cells should the same foreign invader return.

The macrocosm also reflects the microcosm. The Cayce readings compare us to cells, stating that we, as souls, are corpuscles (or cells) of God. What are our needs? What is required for us to attune to God? Can we then extrapolate those needs to the cells in our body?

Abraham Maslow, a noted psychologist, studied twenty-six individuals whom he considered "self-actualized" in an attempt to determine what these very different individuals had in common. From this study, he determined that each of us has a hierarchy of needs:

1. Food, clothing, and shelter.
2. Safety, security, and protection.
3. A sense of belonging, as in a family or a community.
4. Love, affection, and friendship.
5. Dignity, self-respect, and self-esteem.
6. The freedom to create, self-actualization.

To climb the hierarchy, the preceeding level's needs have to be met. If we lived in a ghetto suffering from malnutrition with trash piling high around us, our odds of achieving self-actualization would be lower. Similarly, if we had a speaker in our living room which constantly blared messages of fear or anxiety or just produced jumbled, discordant noise, our progress would also be hindered.

In the same way, the cells of our body require certain conditions to help them in their own attunement process. First, they require the best environment possible. Simply put, they need good nutrition and an environment from which the wastes or toxins have been removed. Second, they need to have the right directions "broadcast" to them by our nervous system and our glands.

Health, then, depends on three key processes—cellular nutrition, tissue drainage, and coordination. When these occur, each cell is free to fulfill its purpose and manifest the promise of life.

The coordination necessary for this to happen occurs at several levels. Like we as humans do, our tissues constantly compete with each other for nourishment and space. Each cell belongs to the whole but shares the most in common with those in his own "house," then "city," then "state," and then "country." Each cell and organ has its own duties, priorities, and survival needs.

Health involves orchestrating these needs for the good of the whole. As Plato observed, "Health is the consummation of a love affair of the organs of the body." Dis-ease and distress can arise when "rebellious forces . . . become as warriors against good . . ." (no. 264–45). The purpose of any therapy is to help the warring influences [become] more aware that they are from the same source. As our parts connect, they automatically self-regulate and begin to work forward with a sense of purpose.

Once this is understood, the purpose of every therapy recommended in the Cayce readings becomes clear. All are intended to help each cell in our body become "self-actualized" so that it can attune to the Divine Source and fulfill its destiny of health.

When this has really been accomplished the sky is the limit! The readings tell us that it is physically "possible for any body to produce [anything] which it has produced before" (no. 2483–1), including teeth or a new limb. Also, as we perfect the receiver, both our mental abilities are enhanced and we manifest the spirit more completely. For most of us, this goal may still be several lifetimes away, but it is obviously still a goal worth pursuing.

As we work with these three bodies, the readings provide certain basic concepts we need to understand. These can be thought of as the readings' "ABCs of Health."

> *"The great end of life is not knowledge but action."*
> THOMAS HENRY HUXLEY

A is for application. The most basic of concepts, it is also one of the most difficult. M. Scott Peck, M.D., in *The Road Less Traveled* refers to laziness—the opposite of application—as the "ultimate original sin, and major impediment to spiritual growth." The Cayce source is clear that Truth becomes a part of our being only as a principle is applied. "The reading itself won't help. It is the application consistently, persistently, conscientiously, prayerfully, that will help the body" (no. 3381–2).

"Hold fast to the center."
TAO TE CHING

B is for balance. "The best is that individual or soul-entity that keeps well balanced, never the extremist . . . And so does it apply in the body forces" (no. 1861–16). The readings compare physical acts of extremism to plunging a white-hot iron into cold water. Just as that leaves scales on the iron, extreme actions with our body leave refuse that must be dealt with. Physiologically, we function best in a range between two comparatively polarized states. Blood pressure can be too high or too low. Hyperglycemia or hypoglycemia occur when the blood sugar deviates from normal. Health involves the balancing of opposites. "In any preventative or curative measure, that condition to be produced is to assist the system to gain its normal equilibrium" (no. 902-1).

"To everything there is a season, and a time for every
purpose under heaven."
ECCLESIASTES 3:1

C is for cycles. Much of the world around us has a rhythmic nature and we are no exception to this ebb and flow of life. Almost every physiological function in our body shows a daily fluctuation—from our temperature to the rate at which our cells regenerate. The readings recognized these rhythms, indicating that the body entirely renews itself in 7-year cycles. Within this larger process, each part of the body has its own unique cycle. The skin completely regenerates every twenty-eight days. This is also the functional cycle of the body's elimination patterns. The liver and spleen are included in those organs that change almost seven times in 7 years.

The exact cycle of function for each organ is dependent on its relationship to the nervous system. Within this cycle, each body system is susceptible to problems at specific points. As a result, a general emotion such as worry can affect various organs, producing different symptoms at different times.

Diagnostically, this is important to remember, as general stressors—such as emotion or poor eliminations—can cause specific problems which may change over time.

Therapeutically, the readings indicate cycles are important because any influence that is given continually to the body causes the portion of the system that normally does that job to lose its activity. Cycling a therapy by alternating it with periods of rest has the opposite effect, causing the body to respond by being more active in that direction.

"Self-discipline is usually love, translated into action."
M. SCOTT PECK, M.D.

D is for discipline. There is a difference between propping up an organism in crisis with medicinal crutches and achieving a cure. True curing of most conditions requires a gentle and continuous coaxing of the body back to center. The readings often emphasize the need for consistency and persistency with any application—often for months or years at a time—to allow time for the body to readjust. Consistency and persistency help to maintain the balance of health. They are also the sisters of patience, something the readings say we all need to learn.

"Man is made by his belief. As he believes, so is he."
BHAGAVAD-GITA

E is for expectancy. The power of belief is enormous. It directly influences the mental patterns creating our physical reality. Any therapy is greatly aided by positive expectancy. Numerous examples of this are given throughout this book. Negative beliefs can be equally powerful and so we need to be careful with the direction of our thoughts. The readings tell us that if we expect much we will obtain much; if we expect nothing, we will obtain nothing. "For what ye ask in His name, believing, and thyself living, ye have already" (no. 3049–1).

"The letter killeth, but the spirit giveth life."
2 CORINTHIANS 3:6

F is for fun. Concepts and disciplines—to help our body—should be liberating, not oppressive. The Cayce readings indicate that it is just as bad to be too health-conscious or addicted to routines as to not do anything at all. Rest and recreation are spiritual, mental, and physical necessities. As we journey towards health, we need to recognize the value of positive emotions, prevent activities from becoming routine, and cultivate the ability to laugh.

Along with these concepts, another generalization needs to be made. While all of us are similar, each of us is "a law unto itself" (no. 902–1). In a room of a hundred people, no two look, speak, or act identically. Each has his or her own personality and characteristics. Our bodies reflect this diversity. The size and shape of each individual's organs are as different as their fingerprints. Stomachs come in an infinite number of variations. So do livers, and spleens, and . . . You name it! Each of us, in this same way, is also biochemically distinct. We have all created different patterns and our bodies reflect this.

This carries several ramifications. First, "What would be beneficial in one for prevention might be harmful to another . . ." (no. 902–1). We have all seen rigorous and clear-eyed older folk who smoke and eat a universally condemned diet and yet continue to thrive. Side effects of medications are another classic example. A drug may resolve one man's high blood pressure while causing another to be impotent and depressed. Penicillin may cure pneumonia or cause a fatal allergic reaction.

Second, this physical diversity applies to us over time as well. "Conditions change from day to day. . . . What may be meat today may be poison tomorrow. That means anybody, too!" (no. 294–121).

Finally, each of us has a "weak link" in our biologic chain. One part wears out first, and when this link breaks, our parts can no longer be held together as a single living being. With a small amount of analysis, we can often identify our own weak links and give them the extra attention they need and deserve.

Take a moment now and consider the individuality of your body. How does your body respond when stressed? Often the most reactive portion will become a weak link. Which portions of your body become ill the most often? Think through the illness patterns of your family—especially those of your parents and grandparents. There are genetic predispositions to certain illnesses which accompany your body. Finally, physical characteristics and weaknesses can be carried across lifetimes. As you identify the weaker links in your chain of health, make the effort to pamper these parts of yourself. Prevention works!

No limitation, including genetics, sets your fate in stone. It merely indicates tendencies. The choice of perpetuating old patterns or choosing a different lifestyle is ever before us.

3

The Dance of Health:
The Place of Illness

. . . the weaknesses in the flesh are the scars of the soul!
EDGAR CAYCE reading no. 275–19

There is set before thee today life and death, choose thou life.
DEUTERONOMY 30:19

A 28-YEAR-OLD FILIPINO-AMERICAN woman, feeling weak and complaining of pain in her joints, visited a clinic in Longview, Washington. Based on the results of blood and urine tests, the physician concluded that the woman was suffering from systemic lupus erythematosus—a disease in which the body's immune system attacks healthy organs with all the ferocity it usually reserves for life-threatening intruders. After various drugs failed to restore her to health, the woman sought the advice of another physician, who confirmed the original diagnosis by examining tissue samples from her kidney. This physician recommended that she follow an aggressive regimen using powerful drugs to dampen the immune system's misguided assault.

Instead, the patient returned to the Philippines where she was treated according to local custom: a witch doctor removed the curse that had been placed on her by a former suitor. Three weeks later she returned to the United States. On re-examination and followup lab studies, she showed none of the symptoms she had displayed earlier. Two years later, she gave birth to a healthy baby girl and continued to remain healthy herself.

This case report was published in the *Journal of the American Medical Association*—not the *National Enquirer*—in 1981. The doctor who reported the case asked his peers: "By what mechanism did the machinations of an Asian medicine man cure" the woman's serious condition? The case and its unexplained happenings raise some interesting questions about the nature of health and illness.

Nationally, we appear to be obsessed with health. Joggers pound the streets in record numbers; diet books are constantly making the bestseller list; and more than 10 percent of our spending goes toward health care, up from 3.5 percent of the gross national product when Cayce was giving his readings. Billions more are spent on "soft" health-care items to give us whiter teeth, less perspiration, hair without dandruff, and a wrinklefree face. Vast sums of money are also spent each year on research.

Despite this outpouring of interest, money, and talent, we do not appear any closer to understanding what health is. Our current approach is firmly rooted in a materialistic philosophy and incorrectly motivated by an overpowering fear of illness and death.

Historically, health has been synonymous with perfection. The word *health* comes from the same root as the word for *wholeness*. This root also gives us the word *holy*, and a traditional prerequisite of holiness has been physical perfection. Many religions have taught that to approach the ultimate reality, the seeker must reflect its perfection as closely as possible. In the Old Testament, Aaron was instructed by God that "he . . . that hath any blemish, let him not approach to offer the bread of his God" (Leviticus 21:17). Similarly, for the Taoists, health is a manifestation of the harmony of heaven on earth. The Nei-Ching, the 4,000-year-old master text of Chinese medicine, refers to ancient sages "who understand Tao, patterned themselves upon the yin and the yang and lived in harmony with the arts of divination . . . thus they could live more than 100 years and remain active without becoming decrepit, because their virtue was perfect and never imperiled." The implication is that health is a reflection of spiritual advancement.

For most of us, however, *perfect* health is very unlikely. Fortunately, health also implies a process. Our bodies exist in a state of dynamic equilibrium, centered somewhere on the continuum from *disease* to *dis-ease* to *ease* to *flour-ease* (flourishing). Along this continuum, we all experience daily swings of the pendulum. Keep track of how you feel for 7 days and you will recognize this phenomenon. One morning you may experience a sore throat. Another day there may be a headache or perhaps just a feeling of heaviness. One study showed that 80 percent of us have some form of temporary physical complaint every single week.

Does this mean that we can never be "healthy?" Not at all. Regardless of our current physical state, each of us can begin to move toward a happier life and positive health. Despite pain, handicaps, or old age, a person can be a living process of wellness. The major prerequisite is an individual's free choice to become a growing, changing person.

The Cayce readings would often ask individuals why they wanted to get better: "What would ye do with thy mind and thy body if they were wholly restored to normalcy in this experience?" (no. 3684–1). As we are able to choose actions of love and spiritual growth in response to this question, we set a course leading to true health at all levels of our being. But "when the body becomes so self-satisfied, so self-centered as to . . . refuse [to] change its attitude . . . there cannot be healing . . ." (no. 3124–2).

To help us with this process, we first need to examine and understand illness and the role it plays in our life. Why do we get sick in the first place? This reflects one of the great philosophical questions: why is there evil in the world? Illness equates to suffering. Surely an omnipotent and all-loving God would not let his or her children suffer in this way.

The answer is that we, not God, have created our illness. Illness *does* carry with it the implication that we are not whole and, as such, it is the carrier of a message to us:

> Hence it may truly be said that to be at-variance [to the divine law] may bring sickness, dis-ease, disruption, distress in a physical body. . . . O that all would gain just that! and not feel, "Yes, I understand—but my desires and my body and my weaknesses—and this or that—and I didn't do it." Who else did?
>
> This may be a hard statement for many, but you will eventually come to know it is true: No fault, no hurt comes to self save that thou hast created in thine consciousness, in thine inner self, the cause. (no. 262–83)

That statement *is* hard to accept. The readings often made it harder by substituting the word *sin* for "at-variance to divine law." The word *sin* has its root in an Anglo-Saxon archery term meaning "off the mark." By stating that "illness is sin," the readings are saying that illness represents evidence that our choices are off the mark from universal law. This can be as simple as making the choice of eating the wrong foods. But the truth is that ". . . there is nothing outside of self half so fearful as that [which] may be builded or brewed within self's own mental and material being" (no. 1928–1).

This tie-in of illness and sin makes most people feel very uncomfortable. One of the most powerful attractions of Pasteur's discovery of bacteria was that disease could be blamed on external forces. It was no longer our fault; those little bugs attacked us. It was part of our uncontrollable destinies. As a society, we are moving away from personal responsibility. Murder is dismissed as temporary insanity. Falling from a ladder becomes the manufacturer's fault and deserving of compensation. Illness must be someone else's fault as well. Our consciousnesses' were soothed by Pasteur's germ-theory, and we chose to ignore his admonition, "The germ is nothing, the soil is everything." Why one person becomes ill while another remains healthy when both are exposed to the same virus was shelved for a later date.

The connection between illness and sin also makes us uncomfortable because we are a judgmental society. We are quick to blame and attach fault and, with it, guilt. A recent *New England Journal of Medicine* editorial (June 1985) argued that the new mind/body approach to cancer should be dropped. A major reason for that position was that too many patients were being made to feel guilty: initially for having the disease in the first place, and then, if they did not improve, for being unable to turn the situation around.

With our current attitude toward illness, the editorial has a point. First, because we approach in fear, death automatically implies failure. It should not. Second, our spirituality is often very judgmental. The message Jesus gave to those gathered around the woman at the well, preparing to stone her, is applicable to how we perceive those around us who are ill. We are all traveling the same journey.

Taking responsibility for our health does not mean getting blamed for the past, but signifies personal involvement in the present. Illness is not a punishment, but it does have significance. If we are spiritual beings—and we are—we would not want it any other way. Illness should play a role in our spiritual pilgrimage. A far worse alternative would be if all our suffering and pain was meaningless and served no purpose.

> For each soul should gain that understanding that whatever may be the experience, if there is not resentment, if there is not contention . . . it is for then that soul's understanding, and will . . . bring the greater understanding of the spiritual in the physical body. (no. 1242–6)

Rather than angrily shout "Why me!", we should quietly ask "Why me?" and search within us for the answer. Illness *can* serve as a teacher, as a feedback loop in our three-dimensional world of cause and effect, and as a purging process to bring us back to God.

Illness may actually present unequaled opportunities for growth. In 1977 the Nobel Prize in chemistry was given to Belgian scientist Ilya Prigogine for his Theory of Dissipative Structures. Prigogine came up with his theory in response to chemistry's Second Law of Thermodynamics, which holds that the universe is running down—everything is going from a higher to lower energy, from organization into chaos. Prigogine showed, using mathematical equations, that while the Second Law holds for the universe as a whole, the process can be reversed under very specific circumstances and an energy system can reorganize into a higher state.

For that to occur, two things are necessary. The first is a dissipative structure. By this, Prigogine means something that consumes energy from the environment and dumps waste back into it. He and the Nobel committee realized that this definition incorporated more than chemicals in the lab: Our bodies qualify and so do our cells. Next, this energy system needs to be placed out of equilibrium, or stressed away from the status quo.

When these two conditions are met, a single stray event can trigger startling consequences. The results can be amplified tremendously and the system can reorganize to a higher level of energy and complexity. In our case, illness can so stress our bodies that it becomes a time of opportunity to reorganize our patterns toward health. "And instead of the conditions . . . becoming stumbling stones to thee, they may become stepping-stones to a larger, a more abundant life of service in His Name" (no. 1452–1).

Take a moment to place this in the perspective of your own life. Reflect on the five most stressful times you have experienced, even if they resulted in "failure." What did you learn from those experiences? Did you turn, or could you have turned, them into stepping stones?

Even with such a perspective, taking responsibility can be tough when we don't understand what is causing our discomfort. All of us understand immediate feedback: when we overeat, our stomach hurts; if we overexercise, our muscles are sore the next day. This direct relationship becomes more difficult to trace, however, in chronic illnesses where cause and effect are subjected to a space-time curvature and a temporal linkage may not always be evident. Symptoms—like images in a dream or metaphors in a poem—can provide feedback and be interpreted at many levels. One individual asked Cayce where and when all her trouble originated. The response was that it began about thirty-five thousand years ago. Just because a beginning is not obvious does not mean that one does not exist.

A valuable place to start our search for the cause of our physical symptoms is in our habits. Pythagoras said, "Man, by his habits, sets into motion those agencies which eventually destroy him."

Despite its hesitancy to do so, medicine now recognizes that many diseases do, in fact, have strong behavioral components as their cause. The top four killers in our country are heart disease, cancer, strokes, and accidents. Diet, smoking, or alcohol consumption plays a role in each of these, prompting a previous surgeon general to observe that it is our lifestyle which is killing us.

What are habits and where do they reside? Our habits are nothing more than the patterns by which we live, formulas from which we react to our world. By definition, a habit causes us to follow a set behavior before investigating whether such a course is wise. Many of these patterns serve us well. We usually drive by reaction, freeing our consciousness to think about other things while we travel. Of course, we sometimes head in directions we hadn't originally intended—to work, for example, when we meant to go to the store. Conditioning like this can also get us in trouble. For example, many of our subconscious driving patterns would place us (as American drivers) in danger in England, where the traffic direction is reversed.

Our body is prone to habit as well. The power of physiological conditioning became obvious with Pavlov's famous experiment at the turn of the century. Every time his dogs were given meat, which naturally made them salivate, a bell was rung. After a period of time, the dogs would salivate just to the sound of the bell.

The entire body, down to the cells of our immune system, appears to be open to such conditioning. In the 1970s Dr. Robert Ader at the University of Rochester demonstrated this by injecting rats with an immunosuppressant drug called cyclophosphamide and adding saccharin to their drinking water. Soon, the taste of saccharin alone suppressed the rats' immune systems.

In another fascinating study, volunteers with known positive reactions to a tuberculin skin test were given this test for 5 months in a row. Each month they came to the same room, with the same furniture, and the same nurse. Each time, there was a red vial with the tuberculin and a green vial with a salt solution which were always injected into the same arms. Each month, these volunteers reacted to the tuberculin with a red swollen skin patch. On the sixth month, the vial's contents were switched without their knowledge. The result? As a group, the volunteers had almost no reaction to the tuberculin. They had been conditioned that the green vial would not produce a reaction and this was sufficient to depress their immune systems' response to the tuberculin.

This type of physiological conditioning constantly affects the way we react to the world. It takes only one or two episodes of anxiety that can be related to a specific event—like public speaking, taking an exam, or sitting in bumper-to-bumper traffic late for an appointment—for us to respond in this same fashion the next time we find ourselves in a similar situation, even if we are not threatened the second time. The conditioning establishes a physiological memory circuit.

An analogy can be made to a multideck tape recorder. Next to this tape recorder sits a large stack of cassette tapes—each labeled for any given situation we might encounter. As we respond to different situations, each of us flips from one tape to another. As the expression goes, "You pushed my button"; in goes a cassette and we play out a certain set of behaviors and thoughts without having really made a conscious decision to do so. We think, speak, feel, and act from that particular tape. Our emotions are inextricably tied into this tape system as well.

What is the anatomical equivalent to this tape deck? Where are these physiological memory circuits of emotion? Psychologists can't agree exactly where they start, the mind or the body. The two oldest psychological theories of emotion serve to illustrate the difference. Walter Cannon argued that emotions originate in the mind. From there, the message is transmitted through the nervous system to the organs of the body to produce the changes in their activity. In other words, if we see a bear in the woods, we say "I am scared" and the message is transmitted to our organs, resulting in rapid pulse and respirations and blood shift from the organs to the muscles. Put more simply, we laugh because we are happy, cry because we are sad, and tremble because we are afraid. The body changes in response to the mind.

In direct contrast to this position is a theory developed independently by the great Harvard psychologist William James and Carl Lange, a Scandinavian. Their theory states that a given event automatically sets off a pattern of bodily changes. The brain then recognizes this pattern as belonging to a specific emotion and labels it as such. Using the example of the bear in the woods, the sight of the animal sets off certain changes governing our heart, respirations, and muscles. These signals then reach the brain and, in a flash, we realize that we are afraid. In other words, we feel happy because we laugh, sad because we cry, and afraid because we tremble.

The first theory states the pattern is in the mind and is translated to the body by the autonomic nervous system. The second says the patterns are in the body and are picked up by the autonomic nervous system and communicated to the mind. Central to both ideas is the autonomic nervous system and this is where the Cayce readings focus their attention, holding it as the critical fulcrum in this whole process.

The readings indicate that habit formation takes place in the subconscious mind, which as you may recall from Chapter Two is linked by the readings directly to the autonomic nervous system. The sympathetic nervous system, referred to in the Cayce readings as the impulsive or imaginative body, is specified as the home of these memory patterns. With this system, our mind and body are inextricably linked together. Every physiological change in our body is accompanied by a corresponding change in our mental-emotional state. Likewise, every change in our perceptions, attitudes, and emotions is translated by the body into an altered physiology.

Where do these patterns initially originate? The Cayce readings go a step further and equate our habits with an Eastern word, *karma*. Stating that this means nothing more than science's cause and effect, or religion's destiny of the soul, its essence is that we must each meet that which we have built. Its value to us lies in its blend of the scientific and religious concepts of where our habits, or patterns, may have originated. It helps us to consider past lives as a possibility, and to consider that current patterns may be the result of choices we made during such past lives. For example, one woman was told that she was allergic to substances which she had misused in a previous lifetime. Similarly, a boy having difficulty with bedwetting was told that this resulted from his having participated in the dunking of witches in Salem, Massachusetts. Not all karma is so distant or romantic, however, as seen in the following interchange:

> Q: Since all disease is caused by sin, exactly what sin causes the colon and elimination condition?
>
> A: The sin of neglect. Neglect is just as much sin as grudge, as jealousy . . . (no. 3051–7)

The pattern of neglecting our bodies in this lifetime is not glamorous, but its effects are just as real.

Let's return to the question, "Why do we want to get well in the first place?" If illness is to serve a meaningful role in our lives, we cannot be content with returning to the same patterns which made us ill in the first place. If we are content, the promise is that we will meet the pattern over and over again until we change it. In this spirit, Jesus is quoted as telling those he healed, "Go and sin no more." In other words, go and change the pattern which has placed you out of harmony in the first place: use illness as the transforming process it is meant to be.

In the struggle to survive a stressful situation, a new way of being often emerges that is much more satisfying than the old. Every culture and religion employ the archetypes of death and rebirth when discussing change and growth. Easter and Passover, symbolic of death and a rebirth into greater freedom, are metaphors for our escape from past conditioning and outmoded patterns of being. The tender, young plant that emerges from a dying seed and the phoenix that arises from its ashes are variations on the theme that life is a continuous process of growth. History is filled with examples of people who have experienced some form of personal transformation as the result of a serious disease or a crippling injury. Helen Keller is such an example. When we are able to use every experience as a tool for self-exploration and growth, then we are well on our way to health. The body may lag behind, even by a lifetime (remember, the physical is the result), but that is inconsequential. Real healing has begun.

And herein lies the beauty of the memory circuits found in the autonomic nervous system. We can "correct habits by forming others! That's everybody!" (no. 475–1). The autonomic nervous system *is* a conditionable system. Every time we access a memory, there is the potential to work with it. We can either reinforce that memory pattern—consciously or unconsciously—or we can begin with the process of extinguishing it by choice. At any given moment, we *can* choose from any of our tapes.

Habits tend to persist, however, unless we move toward a greater self-awareness and consciously choose to change our patterns. To continue growing, life must be characterized by such action and not merely by habitual reaction. Henry Ford noted that "those people who think they can do something and those who think they can't are both right." The next two chapters will help you realize that *there are* tools to help you accomplish your desired transformation.

4

Patterns for Life: Spiritual Tools for Health

. . . healing of the physical without the change in the mental and spiritual aspects brings little real help to the individuals in the end.

EDGAR CAYCE reading no. 4016–1

You ought not attempt to cure the eyes without the head, or the head without the body, so neither ought you attempt to cure the body without the soul.

PLATO

UNTIL THE MID-1970's, science believed that much of the internal workings our body acted independently of our control. We now know that organs can learn to perform various tasks, just as we once learned to walk or ride a bicycle. We can raise or lower blood pressure, change heart rate, alter brain waves, and even teach kidneys to change the rate at which they form urine. We are now discovering that even the immune system is within reach. This marks a big difference between our hardware and that of a computer counterpart—*we can* learn to reprogram ourselves. If our habits are killing us, we can change them.

This sounds simple enough. But there is still a deep mystery as to how these pattern changes can be accomplished. We cannot change a habit by simply voicing the desire and intent. The process is quite different than moving our hand. Our physiological memory circuits are stored in a place that is hard for the cells lying in the thin strips of our brain cortex, to reach.

There is probably good reason for this. As the medical philosopher Lewis Thomas puts it, he would rather be told to take over the controls of a Boeing 747 at 40,000 feet than be told he is in direct control of the approximately five hundred functions his liver performs. He is, he states, "considerably less intelligent than [his] liver."

However, the reaction patterns within our glands and neurons already *do* influence the functioning of our organs. If those messages spell patterns of illness, they require our attention.

The Cayce readings tell us that a higher soul controls habits, rather than being controlled by them. If we agree, we appear to have two choices. The first is to try to determine the spiritual, mental, and physical patterns causing our problems; then work to change them. This is the way to karmically face our patterns. Buckminster Fuller captured the essence of this approach when he said, "Whatever humans have learned had to be learned as a consequence only of trial-and-error experience. Humans have learned only through their mistakes."

The Cayce material outlines a theology which says such an approach is not only the slow way, it also has always ended in failure. It seems we are slow learners; despite our various lifetimes, we have just not caught on. As a result, a second path has been paved for us. Jesus became the Christ and manifested the perfect pattern on the earth. With his death, the curtain secluding the Holy of Holies was torn in half, symbolic of new access routes to God. No longer is God to be found as the cloud or the burning bush; instead God is within, awaiting us. Practically speaking, our patterns have been placed within our reach to change without having to karmically face them.

This concept is expressed in the word *grace*.

There appear to be at least two ways to work with grace.

The New Testament teaches that grace comes as a gift from God, the result of our faith. It is not earned through our own efforts. This is the essence of the first path. "There is grace through the power of the belief . . . in the divine" (no. 3249–1).

We know that belief alone can create powerful changes in our physiology. Two thousand years ago, a woman touched the hem of Jesus' garment and was healed of prolonged uterine bleeding. The Christ explained that her faith had made her whole. A dramatic negative example of this can be seen in the cultural practice of voodoo. There have been many documented cases of death attributed to voodoo. In each case, the victim was both aware of the spell and a firm believer in its power.

Another example of the power of expectancy involves the phenomenon of false pregnancies, known medically as pseudocyesis. In such cases, through the woman's belief that she is with child, her breasts enlarge and become tender, her abdomen enlarges at the normal rate for pregnancy, and there may be the secretion of milk. Some women have even experienced sensations of fetal movement. A famous example of this phenomena is a "pregnancy" experienced by Mary Tudor in the sixteenth century. It lasted 9 months and ended with two episodes of false labor.

Faith healing depends on belief as well. In his book *Persuasion and Healing: A Comparative Study of Psychotherapy*, Jerome Frank, M.D., cites an experiment done in the 1950s that involved three hospitalized women. One woman was dying of metastatic cancer, another had a chronic gall bladder problem, and the third was having great difficulty recovering from abdominal surgery and "was practically a skeleton." The doctor of the three women asked a well-known local faith healer to try healing them from a distance. The faith healer went to work, without the doctor telling his patients. Nothing happened. The physician then told the women about the healer and said that the healer would attempt to help them from a distance on a certain day and time. This time the healer did nothing. At the stated time, all three women were noted to improve dramatically. The woman with the gall bladder problem suddenly felt better, was able to go home, and remained symptom-free for several years. The surgical patient was permanently cured. And the cancer patient recovered sufficiently from severe anemia and fluid retention to go home and resume running her household. She had no further symptoms until her death.

Belief is often strengthened by an external stimulus, be it the mention of a healer or the use of a pill. In the late 1950s, Dr. Bruno Klopfer was participating in trials of a new drug, Krebiozen, that was being touted as a miracle cancer cure. One patient with an advanced lymphoma involving the immune system responded amazingly well to the drug. His cancerous growths "melted away like snowballs." Several months later, newspapers reported the drug had been discredited and was considered ineffective. The patient's tumors promptly returned.

Dr. Klopfer, suspecting the patient's belief was responsible for his initial "cure," told the patient he had obtained a newly made, more potent form of the drug. He then treated the patient with only distilled water. The tumors once again melted away. Several months later, definitive studies were published showing that Krebiozen was worthless. The tumors rapidly reappeared and the patient died shortly thereafter.

Using the model of our patterns as cassette tapes, belief can offer a dramatic way of changing the existing tape in the tape deck. Inserting a tape of hope or confidence will result in physiological changes that will facilitate healing. At the other extreme a harmful belief—voodoo practices, for example—can create a physiology which blocks healing and may destroy us. The Cayce readings advised one surgeon that the greatest help he could provide to his patients was his ability to help them create positive beliefs:

> . . . the personality of arousing hope, of creating confidence, of bringing the awareness of faith into the consciousness of an individual is very necessary. . . . Thus the entity may through the use of the abilities as a conversationalist . . . bring great help, much more than through the use of drugs or the scalpel. (no. 5083–2)

Most physicians are not fully aware of the power belief has in the healing process. Consequently, they rarely use it to fullest advantage. One reading said that a person could be injected with one thing and be told it was something else and their body would most likely respond as if the imagined substance was real.

Experimentation has verified this. Another experiment cited by Dr. Frank in his book *Persuasion and Healing* involved a woman with morning sickness. The woman was told she was going to receive a powerful drug to relieve nausea. Instead, she was given Ipecac, a drug used in emergency rooms to cause people who have ingested a poison to vomit and had previously been shown to produce nausea and vomiting in her. After receiving the Ipecac, the woman reported that her nausea had improved. A measuring device placed in her stomach objectively confirmed the fact that her stomach was not responding to the medication. This woman's power of belief was stronger than the drug. For doctors, who are proud of their recent alliance with science, this seems too much like magic. Most are unwilling to blend the best of both worlds.

Healing as the result of belief, however, is not always permanent. Many ailments require a longer healing period than the relatively brief time of altered physiology offered by a faith experience. Jerome Frank, M.D., the doctor interested in the power of belief, notes that "no one has ever regrown an amputated limb at Lourdes." Faith healings appear to lie within the constraints of our physiology and the necessary depth of belief is difficult to sustain for a prolonged period. Reverting back to the old tapes is easy to do.

There is a second path to grace. This approach can help sustain a physiology of faith and, over time, actually change the tapes with which we respond to a given situation. The techniques of this second path shake up the tape deck, the autonomic nervous system (ANS). Compatible with Ilya Prigogine's Theory of Dissipative Structures, when the ANS is "stressed" or its normal balance altered, the opportunity is present to work directly on our tapes.

Research shows that the extensive memory patterns in our subconscious rarely change in response to direct commands. These memories, however, become much more accessible in physiological states produced by the disruption of our normal autonomic balance. This concept forms the basis for most mind/body healing therapies. There are numerous methods which can produce these changes. These techniques are incorporated into the fabric of all religions and society as a whole. Both Zen Buddhist meditators and tribal dancers employ them. Let's examine why they work.

All of these techniques rely on their ability to manipulate the ANS away from its normal equilibrium. The balance of the ANS is controlled by the hypothalamus, a portion of our brain that is the size of a small prune and lies just above the pituitary. Having extensive connections with other areas of the brain, the hypothalamus is thought to act as *the* communication switchboard between our mind and body. In this capacity, it serves as a regulator of the endocrine glands and immune system, in addition to the ANS.

In the 1940s, Swiss Nobel laureate Walter Hess discovered that the stimulation of different areas of an animal's hypothalamus can produce diametrically opposed physiological states. One state involves a heightened activity level which resembles the "fight-or-flight" response, and causes, among other things, the heart to beat faster, blood pressure to rise, and sweat glands to go into overdrive. Stimulating another part of the hypothalamus can quiet the entire body, leading to decreased muscle tone, a slowed heart rate, and sleeplike brain waves—all combining to produce a state of deep rest and relaxation. In terms of the ANS, these changes represent deviations from the normal resting balance. In the first state, the sympathetic nervous system becomes dominant, while the latter physical changes occur with dominance of the parasympathetic nervous system.

As we've noted, disrupting the ANS equilibrium in either direction appears to open the tape deck and provide access to changing the tapes. Closely linked with such physiological changes are experiences of altered states of consciousness. Our usual physical consciousness, housed in the outer cortex of our brain, is quieted, and mystical states have been experienced at both ends of this autonomic spectrum.

A number of cultural and religious practices incorporate these altered states to create or change our memory patterns. Examples involving sympathetic nervous system dominance include the circling dances of the Sufi whirling dervishes and the prolonged shouting and violent abdominal contractions of Ishiguro Zen practitioners. In the West, charismatic church services and healings also incorporate these states. In American society, many of the rituals which we have created to mark life passages trigger sympathetic nervous system dominance as well, and this may help us to adapt to new patterns of living. Events such as weddings are often large affairs "to make the family happy"; however, they also can activate the fight-or-flight system.

An equal number of religious and cultural practices involve quieting the sympathetic nervous system and energizing the parasympathetic nervous system. Meditation, hypnosis, progressive muscle relaxation, biofeedback, and candlelight ceremonies are examples of this.

Can the effects of meditation on our memory circuits really be compared to the whoops and screams of a war dance? The Cayce readings say yes. The difference is that the changes produced by the latter result in a negative outcome, while the other has a positive spiritual purpose.

A similar dichotomy exists in the two major ways psychology approaches treating a phobia; in other words, the two methods used to change a specific fear tape. One, implosion therapy, involves confronting a person directly with his fear. If a person is scared of spiders, he is shown movie after movie of spiders. He then graduates to looking at real spiders, and continues progressively working with them until he can hold a spider in his hand. As you can imagine, the fight-or-flight response is elicited during this therapy.

The second technique is known as systematic desensitization. This method teaches a phobic individual to thoroughly relax or quiet his sympathetic nervous system, allowing the parasympathetic nervous system to become dominant. Then and only then, he is told to think of spiders, but only until he feels the slightest tinge of anxiety. At that point, he should remove spiders from his mind and work at relaxing again. This continues until he is able think of spiders without feeling anxiety. Then, like the first method, the degree of contact with spiders is progressively increased.

Both techniques work. Both obviously allow access to the tape labeled "reaction to spiders."

In choosing between the two extremes of autonomic imbalance, most religions teach that the safer path is quieting the system. The Cayce material concurs. Meditation tops the list of the readings' suggested techniques for pursuing spiritual growth and change. The readings say that *all* of us eventually have to learn to meditate, just as we once had to learn to walk.

The readings define meditation as attuning our mental and physical bodies to their spiritual source. As opposed to prayer in which we speak to God, meditation is an activity in which God speaks to us. Through consistent practice, we not only can rearrange our tapes, but we also alter the glandular patterns creating our dispositions and character. *The Secret of the Golden Flower*, a Taoist text of meditation, says that the daily practice of a 20-minute meditation can save us ten thousand lives. The Bible tells us that "he that dwelleth in the secret place of the most High shall abide under the shadow of the Almighty" (Psalms 91:1).

There are a number of meditative techniques. The method suggested by the readings is simple and easy to learn. Start by choosing a regular time of day for meditation. Your body will come to expect this time and you may find it easier to focus and quiet your mind. Setting aside a regular time will also help you to remember to meditate. A 15- to 20-minute block of time is a good starting period.

Next, choose aids to help you attune and relax before you meditate. This is a personal decision. Ideas that people have found helpful include: listening to relaxing or inspirational music, chanting and/or breathing exercises, head and neck exercises (described in Chapter Nine), incense, and reading from the Bible or other holy books.

As you prepare to enter the silence, sit in a straight-back chair or lie on your back. Keep your spine as straight as possible. If you are lying down, join your hands over your solar plexus. Rest them on your lap if you are sitting.

Begin with a few moments of prayer. The readings say the Lord's Prayer has a special symbology which reawakens patterns conducive to meditation, making it especially appropriate. A personal prayer is also effective. If you are not able to quiet your being and you continue to feel anxiety, anger, or fear, spend the remaining time in prayer and do not continue.

After your prayer, repeat an affirmation or phrase which reflects your highest guiding principle. Try to feel the meaning of the words. As you feel uplifted, stop repeating the words and silently concentrate on the inner spirit they have created. Continue until you notice that your attention has been distracted by other thoughts. Don't worry, this is normal. Bless whatever comes to your mind and then release it. Gently come back to your affirmation and repeat the process. These moments of uplifted silence form the core of meditation: "The Lord is in His holy temple: let all the earth keep silence before Him" (Hebrews 2:20).

As you finish, disperse the energy you have raised unselfishly by closing your meditation with a prayer for others. Unless they have made a specific request of you, surround the individuals for whom you are praying with the presence of the Christ and bless them.

Another technique strongly suggested by the Cayce readings is the presleep suggestion. This is especially effective with children. The readings indicate that the time immediately before and as we drift into sleep is ideal for gaining access to the internal tape deck. This method is recommended for a variety of physical and mental problems. As we enter sleep, many of the same physiological changes occur as when we meditate. Our brain waves and heart rate slow. Our respiration slows and becomes even and our blood pressure is lowered. Our sympathetic nervous system is quieted.

When we directly work with our patterns like this, it is important to use a constructive approach. As noted earlier, the readings recommend beginning every meditation with an uplifting phrase. Similarly, presleep suggestions should be worded in an affirming, positive manner, not as a command to not do something.

We usually assume techniques like meditation and presleep suggestions are safe, but they can carry some risk. Material related to the readings warns that without proper precautions, "the opening of the door between the physical and the spiritual will result in turmoil within, striking at the weakest point." This is a strong statement. We usually think of meditation as capable of only producing good. The case of one woman who obtained a reading emphasizes this warning. She listed numerous complaints, including buzzing in her ears, difficulty hearing, frequent headaches, a feeling of dullness, depression, and occasional abnormal functioning of her kidneys, liver, and lungs. Her reading indicated that these occurred because she was meditating when she was anxious and not physically ready to meditate.

A study comparing persons who practiced Transcendental Meditation (TM) daily to others who had dropped out of the initial meditation training course reached a similar conclusion. The researchers looked at such factors as depression, frustration, restlessness, withdrawal, suspiciousness, and confusion. The study found that 46 percent of the meditators had an increase in one of these symptoms as compared to 19 percent in the group that had chosen not to meditate. This doesn't mean we should not meditate, but it does mean we need to be careful about what we dwell on while we meditate.

Meditation and similar techniques merely open our tape decks so we can work with the tapes. They have no effect on what we do once we get into the system. One reading offers the hypothetical example of a person influenced *only* by his or her meditations. The reading states that if fed only spiritual material for 7 years, the person could become a light to the world. If fed only material things, he or she would become a Frankenstein with no concept of the spiritual. We need to know and to specify the direction we want to go *before we begin*. Remember Alice's query in *Through the Looking Glass*: "Would you tell me, please, which way I ought to go from here?" The answer applies to us as well: "That depends a good deal on where you want to get to . . ."

The critical task for each of us is to know the guiding principle behind our conscious and our unconscious choices. The Cayce readings name this principle "the ideal." The readings further say that establishing an ideal is *the* most important thing we can do. Before we go and play with our tapes, we must give direction to their replacement. This applies equally to the tapes which give us a colon condition and to those which keep us in a state of anger. "Healing for the physical body, then, must be first the correct choice of the spiritual import held as the ideal of the individual" (no. 2528–2). The readings strongly recommend that each of us take the time to write down our ideal.

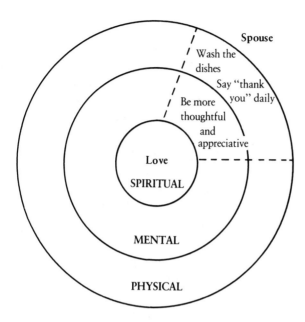

Figure 4-1. Ideals chart.

An effective tool to help is the chart in Figure 4-1. The first step is to choose a single word that most closely describes your spiritual ideal at this moment. This should be the word that awakens *the highest* in you. This may be a word like *love, service, Jesus,* or *Buddha.* It is, and it should be, very personal. It may change as you grow and develop. Once you have chosen this word, write it down in the small center circle.

Next, identify the different areas of your life in which you expend the most time and energy. Examples might include spouse or family, job, friends/neighbors, God/church, and self. Divide the two outer circles into this number of pie-shaped segments. The middle circle will now relate to your mental ideal in each of these areas, the outermost circle to your physical ideal.

As you work with the mental ideal, the guiding question should be: "*As I say the word I have chosen as my spiritual ideal, what comes to mind as the attitude which should govern my interactions here?*"

As an example, if a person's spiritual ideal is *love*, then his or her mental ideals may include being thoughtful and appreciative toward his or her spouse.

In the same way, work with the physical ideal for each aspect of your life. Instead of attitudes, the object now is to think about actions. The guiding question might be: "*What can I do to manifest my spiritual and mental ideals in this area of my life?*" To continue with the above example, that person may choose to wash the dishes daily or say "thank you" to their spouse at least twice a day.

Writing your ideal down is the first step; next is placing it in action. "For as ye apply them they become thy ideals. To be just as theories they do not belong to thee . . . It's the application of same that counts" (no. 5091–3).

Another technique to access one's tapes is hypnosis. Hypnosis involves a simple shifting of consciousness from a waking state to a subconscious place which can be useful therapeutically. Done properly, it can produce the same relaxed and refreshed feeling you might get after a good night's sleep or meditation.

Many books and films unfortunately have created a multitude of misconceptions about hypnosis. Contrary to popular opinion, hypnosis cannot be imposed against one's will. The subject remains completely aware, has total control over each step of the process, and cannot be *made* to do anything. This does not, however, make it completely safe.

The readings recommend hypnosis in approximately 50 percent of the instances it is mentioned, and warn against it—sometimes strongly—in the other 50 percent. Inconsistent? No. The hesitancy is because this technique also opens the tape deck. It differs from meditation, however, because another individual—the hypnotist—manipulates the tapes with his or her hypnotic suggestion. The readings imply that a hypnotized individual can be affected by the spoken words of the hypnotic suggestion *and* the character and disposition of the hypnotist. Therefore, a hypnotist with high ideals is very important.

Just as effective and potentially safer is the use of self-hypnosis (which is what actually occurs within the hypnotic process; a trained therapist merely acts as a facilitator). A tape-recorded induction can be just as effective as a "live" induction. Homemade tapes, which are easy to prepare, can be personalized and aimed at any type of problem/opportunity.

Such a tape usually has three components: the induction guiding you into self-hypnosis, a middle section of positive suggestions and directed visualization exercises, and a wake-up procedure. In general, the subconscious responds best to vivid visual imagery, not to direct commands. The suggestion that one's arm is feeling as light as a feather or has helium balloons attached to it works better than the direction "Raise your arm." Books are available which can guide you through recording your own tape.

A final important technique is working with dreams. This is one way in which the keeper of the tapes, the subconscious, speaks to our physical consciousness. Dreams always tell us something about ourselves. Remember: when you dream, you write the script, cast the players, and design the set. Dreams can provide clues to the unconscious factors and patterns that affect our health; factors which we might otherwise ignore. The Talmud says that a dream which is not understood is like a letter which is not opened.

We do not usually associate the techniques discussed in this chapter with physical healing. They do not seem as concrete or as practical as a spinal manipulation or a castor oil pack. The Cayce material is clear, however, that our spiritual and mental patterns create the person we find ourselves to be. Addressing these patterns and transforming them, where necessary, *are* vital steps on our journey to health.

5

Taming the Wild Horses:
Working with Emotions

The organs weep the tears the eyes refuse to shed.
SIR WILLIAM OSLER

*Worry and fear [are] the greatest foes to [a] normal healthy
physical body. . . .*
EDGAR CAYCE reading no. 5497–1

HE TOOK HER IN his arms again and drew her to him, and suddenly she became small in his arms, small and nestling. It was gone,
and she began to melt in a marvellous peace. And as she melted small
and wonderful in his arms, she became infinitely desirable to him, all
his blood-vessels seemed to scald with intense yet tender desire, for
her, for her softness, for the penetrating beauty of her in his arms,
passing into his blood."

This love passage, written by D. H. Lawrence in 1928, illustrates
a point: "For, thoughts are things! and they have their effect upon
individuals . . . just as physical as sticking a pin in the hand!" (no.
386-2). Reading such passages will dilate the pupils, get the heart
pumping a little quicker, and activate the sweat glands, even if just
slightly.

Our thoughts will activate the appropriate tape in our subconscious memories. The resulting physical changes are real. Imagining an action creates the same physiology as doing the action. Studies have shown that mentally obsessing on something stressful can affect the body more than experiencing it. Jesus made reference to this in the Sermon on the Mount when he taught that anger or lust are no different than murder or adultery.

The patterns in place now are helping or blocking our health at this moment. Meditation and similar techniques work, but the changes occur slowly. The readings speak of a complete change taking 7 years. The question arises, "What am I supposed to do right now?" There *are* activities we can do today to deal with current habits while we're waiting for the longer-term changes to take place.

One way we experience the tapes already in place is through our emotions. The readings state that emotions originate from the connection of mind and spirit. The way we experience emotions, however, is through the physiology they create. It is because of our physical bodies that we are able to experience the sensations of anger, jealousy, and ecstasy. And it is from the physical changes that such emotions produce that we become aware of our bodies. Our emotions are a major component of our "psychosomatic networks," or mind/body networks. As a result, emotions play a major role in our feedback learning systems. They also are part of the reason for our entrapment in the material world: we want to physically experience feelings.

There is no doubt that emotions have a strong physical component. Our feelings are the product of millions of neurologic and biochemical processes occurring within us.

The Cayce readings tell us that "The emotions . . . are as electronic energies. . . . [leaving] the blood . . . *with* a glow from the emotions controlled through the centers or lines of the nervous systems for both positive and negative natures" (no. 263-13). The term "electronic energies," interpreted in the light of quantum mechanics, is descriptive of molecules circulating in the blood.

Science is confirming that this is the case. Let me give you an example. Neuropeptides are small protein molecules (electron energies) found throughout the body. Their activity is most concentrated in our limbic system, the part of the brain that has been linked with emotions. Valium and other mood-altering drugs act at these same limbic sites. Like Valium, the activity of the neuropeptides helps determine the "mind state" we are in. As it turns out, the rest of the body has receptors for these molecules as well, and at the same time they are altering our consciousness they are also affecting the working of our organs.

For example, imagine you've been strolling along the beach in the summertime. The sun has been beating down, you haven't had water to drink for hours, and you've become dehydrated. The internal events start when the kidneys sound the alarm by releasing some of these neuropeptides. When the neuropeptides reach the brain, a chemical cascade of molecules spreads through the body, causing it to act as a whole. Blood vessels constrict, kidneys stop producing urine, and the limbic system sends a message to your brain's outer cortex, producing the thought, "Hey, I'm thirsty. I'd do anything for a glass of water."

Another research area which explores the physiology of our emotions is the new field of psychoneuroimmunology. The name is a mouthful, but the concept is simple. The mind (psycho), through the nervous system (neuro), affects the behavior of the immune system (immunology). Just 10 years ago, the best immunologists in the country would have questioned the validity of this idea because white blood cells seem to work just fine isolated from the nervous system in a laboratory petri dish. They seemed to be "worlds unto themselves." Research in the last few years has shown conclusively that this just isn't so. Many experiments in the field of psychoneuroimmunology have shown that immune function is affected by our emotional states. People who are grieving, depressed, or otherwise stressed—be they medical students approaching an exam or recent widowers—have impaired immune functioning. At the other end of the spectrum, medical students who viewed a film of Mother Teresa and her inspirational work showed increased production of salivary antibodies which protect against germs.

Since our immune systems play a role in defending us against infectious diseases and cancer and in the development of autoimmune diseases and allergies, this connection could eventually be found to have major ramifications. Every single communication system in the body which has been looked at to date affects the immune system, including the neuropeptides mentioned above.

Two classic pathways that chart how our bodies respond to stress are known to play major roles in this communication (see Figure 5-1).

Hans Selye proposed the existence of a "general adaptation syndrome" after finding that stress always produced the same changes in the animals he was studying—the adrenal glands enlarged, the thymus and other lymphatic tissue shrunk, and gastrointestinal ulceration occurred. Recognizing these changes were the tip of the iceberg, Selye went on to state, "Virtually every organ and every chemical constituent of the human body is involved in the general stress reaction." He found that these changes start with signals from the hypothalamus, the control center described in Chapter Four, directing the pituitary to influence the entire endocrine system, especially the adrenal glands.

Walter Cannon in 1929 described another patterned response of the body to stress—the previously mentioned fight-or-flight response. The name was chosen because of Cannon's conjecture that this response was useful to our ancestors in dealing with the environmental stressors of their time—such as walking around a rock and finding a saber-toothed tiger. It involves an outpouring of flow along our sympathetic nervous system which causes the release of adrenalin and the constriction of our blood vessels. This results in increased blood pressure, heart rate, breathing rate, energy production, and flow of blood to the muscles. These actions increase the chance of success whether the caveman chose to fight the tiger or turn in flight. However, in today's world, when we are upset with our boss, the options do not include striking him or her, or running away. Our immune systems—and the rest of our body—take the beating instead.

Has this understanding of how emotions affect us produced any dramatic findings? No. The most important contribution to date has

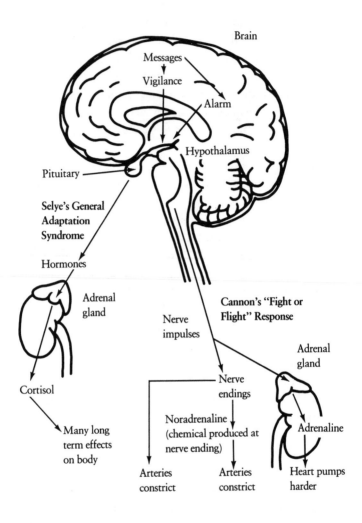

Figure 5-1. How the "general adaptation syndrome" and the "fight or flight" response affect the body.

been that there is now good hard data—the kind science likes—showing connections between our thoughts and emotions and the workings of our bodies. Numerous studies now demonstrate what is common sense and has been known by observation alone for thousands of years—"good" emotions help our bodies to work better and negative emotions can eventually destroy us. The readings are filled with similar wisdom:

> Anger causes poisons to be secreted from the glands. Joy has the opposite effect. (no. 281–54)
>
> No one can hate his neighbor and not have stomach or liver trouble. No one can be jealous and allow the anger of same and not have upset digestion or heart disorder (no. 4021–1)
>
> The thoughts of the body act upon the emotions as well as the assimilating forces. Poisons are accumulated or produced by anger or by resentment or animosity. (no. 23–3)
>
> Hate, malice, and jealousy only create poisons within the minds, souls, and bodies of people. (no. 3312–1)

What does all this mean? To date, much has been made of the damage that stress can do to our bodies. In fact, stress has been emphasized so much that a fear of stress has been produced. We now are fearing fear and compounding the problem. Often we ignore the fact that stress is produced by *our* reaction to a given situation—a particular tape playing itself out. We can choose to change the tape that gets inserted into the tape deck, often handling the same situation in a manner which does not create these changes of fear in our bodies.

The key is to manage stress, not necessarily to avoid it. Hans Selye pointed out that stress can be the spice of life. Adversity presents opportunities which can forge the spirit. If we are able to reframe a situation as a challenge instead of a threat, we will have a different physical response.

Several examples will help illustrate this. First, a study published in *Science* in August of 1983 showed that a sense of control over a situation changes the physiological response. Experiments were conducted in which two sets of rats were exposed to the same type and amount of stressor—a mild electric shock to the tail. One group was given the perception that they had control over when the shocks occurred, while the shocks given the second group were completely random. There was a significant suppression of the cellular immune response only in the latter group. Similar studies published in *Science* in 1979 and 1982 showed that tumor development was enhanced in the "helpless, hopeless" group.

Similar results have been found by Dr. Suzanne Kobassa in studies of businesspeople and executive lawyers. She found that individuals with a great deal of life stress were less affected physically if three attitudes towards life were present. These were a sense of commitment, a sense of control, and a sense of challenge as opposed to alienation, helplessness, and apathy. When the three positive attitudes were present, the individual was found to have a stress-hardy personality which responded to stressful situations by increasing his or her interaction with it, not trying to escape it.

The effects of stress are also greatly buffered by the love and support of other people. Insurance companies have found that men who are kissed good-bye by their wives in the morning have fewer car accidents and live 5 years longer. Two researchers in Israel studied ten thousand men with the risk factors for developing angina pectoris and arrived at a similar conclusion. The most accurate psychological factor in predicting who would develop symptomatic angina was the answer "no" to the question, "Does your wife show you her love?"

More evidence on the power of love was obtained by happenstance in a study conducted at Ohio State University. A group of investigators was studying the effects of a high fat and cholesterol diet in rabbits. At the end of a certain period of time the rabbits' arteries were examined for the presence of atherosclerosis, the plaques which can cause heart attacks and strokes in humans. To their surprise, they found one group of rabbits developed 60 per cent less atherosclerotic changes than the other groups. In reviewing their experimental protocol, they found only one difference between these rabbits and the others. They had been cared for by an investigator who regularly removed them from their cages and petted, stroked, and talked to them. Not believing their findings, the investigators repeated the experiment twice more with the same results.

In the simplest terms, emotions fall into two broad categories, love and fear. "Fear is the root of most of the ills of mankind . . ." (no. 5459–3), while "Perfect love casteth out fear" (1 John 4:18). At each moment of our lives, we are given the choice of which of these states we will choose. Our choice impacts our health in very direct ways.

The first step in consciously working with this choice is to be aware at any given moment of which state we are in. Fear produces a defensive response of our body which can be identified physiologically as a stress reaction—muscles tighten, breathing becomes shallow and irregular, hands become cold and clammy, and our heart may start pounding. Love is associated with the opposite physiological response—giving us a sense of openness, relaxation, and letting go.

A critical step toward health for each of us is to make a conscious choice for the physiology of love and to know what this feels like inside our bodies. Sometimes, we have been tense for so long that this tension has becom our "normal" state. It's possible to go through the day with clenched fists or teeth and not be aware of it until we experience a tension headache or a sore back. Figure 5-2 helps illustrate some of the physiological changes fear can elicit and lists ten common stress-related symptoms.

Take a few moments right now, close your eyes, quiet yourself, and become aware of your body. Check the tension of your jaw by opening and closing your mouth slowly. Do a few head rolls—are your neck and shoulder muscles loose or are they tight and sore? Ask yourself "Where am I tense?" and scan the rest of your body. When you become aware of a tense area, exaggerate the tension slightly by contracting that muscle so you can sense it better. Now check your mouth—is it dry? Become aware of your breathing—is it slow and deep? Check the temperature of your hands—are they cold? Are your palms sweaty? Do you feel calm and relaxed? Anxiety manifests differently in each of us. Become aware of how it affects you and reach the point where you can recognize these signals.

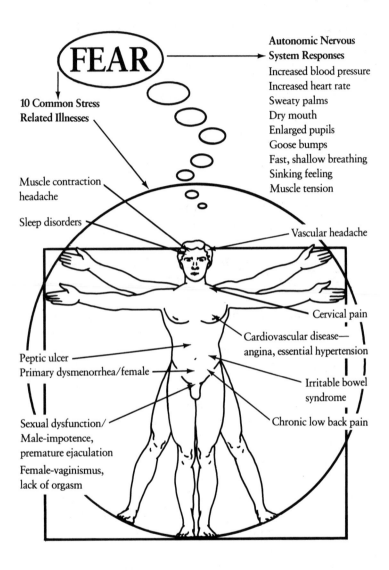

Figure 5-2.   Ways fear can manifest in the body.

When you identify tension, take a moment to visualize it dissipating. "Quiet, meditation, for a half to a minute, will bring strength—will the body see *physically* this *flowing* out to quiet self, whether walking, standing still, or resting" (no. 311–4).

Another simple and effective way to release stored tension is with the use of deep abdominal breaths which incorporate your diaphragm. This helps set a more relaxed resting tone for the autonomic nervous system. The readings recommend breathing in through the left nostril to relax the body and the right nostril for strength. With each breath, exhale slowly through your mouth.

It will be the rare individual who doesn't identify some fear within. As we've noted, this fear has real effects on the body and needs to be dealt with. The following process should be helpful.

First, acknowledge your fear. This involves owning the emotion and being willing to face it directly. The best path away from fear and stress is to confront them directly. Hiding from them or denying their existence strengthens them, fuels the sense of helplessness and the inability to cope, and may exact a heavy price in physical symptoms.

Next, try to find the source of your fear. What is producing that physiological state in your body? Often, it is the result of something or someone continually pushing the button for the tape labeled fear in your sympathetic nervous system. Most commonly, this stimulus takes the form of a relationship or interaction—it does not occur in a vacuum.

Third, when you are able to find a source, work on this aspect of your life. Sometimes this can be done directly; sometimes it needs to be done through the use of prayer and visualization. One useful technique is an exercise that can be done at the end of meditation or prayer. It is specifically intended to help with a difficult relationship.

Spend the first half a minute forgiving yourself for specific things you may have done to create the situation. Then, for a half a minute ask God to forgive your past or present attitude toward this person. Take the next 30 seconds to forgive the other person for any hurt they have inflicted on you. For the last half a minute, pray for the person and bless them. Do this for 28 days and see if you note a change in your attitude toward that person.

If, after sincerely searching, you cannot identify the source of a given emotion, then you should move past it. The key at this point is to realize that every thought is a prayer: To what are you praying? If your thoughts are constantly reverberating with negative emotions, choose to make a change. While that is not easy, it can be done.

One way to do this, according to the readings, is to turn toward the light and place the shadows behind. A story is told about Alexander the Great as a boy which illustrates this point. A magnificent unbroken stallion was brought to his father's court. All the great horsemen of the land attempted to ride the powerful animal but were quickly thrown from his back. Alexander, already a keen observer, noticed the horse was frightened of its own shadow. After getting his father's hesitant permission to attempt a ride, Alexander turned the horse's face into the sun and rode to greatness on the back of his now famous Bucephalus. In the same way, as we are able to focus on the light of the Christ, the shadows causing our fears will fall from our sight and not affect us.

Let me share several methods to help you do this. The first technique is called "thought stopping." This simple tool helps lay aside those thoughts that hamper our health and allows us to substitute higher ones in their place. To employ this, you need to first become an expert on *your* own style of negative thinking. Practice becoming detached from your reactions to a situation and observing yourself. During this initial phase, don't censor your thoughts, just make note of them. Take a week to make a list of the traps you most often fall into. Then devise a list of quick responses—personalized to your own needs—that you can use to replace your negative and unproductive thoughts.

Here are some examples:

- I am a good and loving person.
- I am a child of God.
- Relax. I can manage this situation.
- I can cope.

As soon as you are aware that you are regressing into negative thinking, choose to substitute a positive thought in its place. Do not give the negative thought energy. If a negative thought persists, try a forceful rebuttal statement directed at the negative thought. Here are some examples:

- Stop this helpless stuff.
- No more of this garbage.
- Enough negative stuff.

Always follow a forceful rebuttal with one of the positive thoughts you have chosen to affirm your abilities.

This technique employs your gift of free will to choose what you wish your mind to dwell on. William James, the great psychologist, was in the midst of a severe and prolonged depression early in his life. He describes having a realization that he had total freedom to choose between one thought and another. He chose to release his negative thinking and went on to do great things.

Another technique is visualization. This works with the concept that as we choose thoughts, we directly affect the working of our body. Visualization can be used to positively harness our thoughts to aid us in the healing process.

Our daily imagery affects us more than we realize. When you think of the bumper-to-bumper traffic you face at the end of each day, you unconsciously tighten the muscles of your jaw and neck. When your thoughts turn to your spouse who is making your favorite meal, these muscles will relax. Athletes work creatively with this concept in competition, going over and over their event in their minds before they actually compete.

Visualization employs a technique similar to "thought stopping," but uses pictoral images in place of verbal phrases. Rather than worrying or imagining the worst, we should "see" the body working as well as it can or, as the readings say, "functioning in a way which will bring about that desired" (no. 1048–3).

Both the readings and current literature indicate certain methods will help us accomplish the results we seek with visualization. First, the images should be our own, but should also be based on what we can learn about the anatomy and physiology of the portion of the body we are trying to affect. Next, the images should be as consistent and constant as we can make them. (Remember each thought is a prayer.) Finally, the visualization should be taken to completion each time. It should end with us "seeing" the goal accomplished.

Another technique is based the knowledge that we can affect the way we are feeling by manipulating the muscles of our face. Paul Ekman completed some wonderful research which demonstrated that we can create physiologies of stress and depression or of happiness and relaxation with the use of our eighty facial muscles. Our internal physiology will mirror our facial expressions and we literally feel what we put on our faces. If your face shows sorrow, you'll experience sadness inside. If you can smile through sadness or depression, it will help lift away these emotions and return you to a state of joy.

Similarly, regardless of our mood, our bodies benefit from humor.

> Remember that a good laugh, an arousing even to . . . hilariousness, is good for the body, physically, mentally, and gives the opportunity for greater mental and spiritual awakening. (no. 2647–1)

We can also help others by bringing joy and humor into their lives. The readings encourage setting the goal of bringing laughter into the lives of at least three people a day.

One place that the patterns from our tapes are both readily visible and easily accessible for therapy is in our muscles. Numerous individuals have described the concept of muscles tensing into a body armature in response to emotionally and physically threatening situations. There are now an equal number of techniques that work directly to release this stored tension and help transform our mental patterns. They include rolfing, bioenergetics, and the Alexander and Feldenkrais techniques. Simple massage can also recreate emotional feelings within us as tense areas are worked on. These locations are worth noting and working with directly.

Another technique designed to help elicit relaxation is progressive muscle relaxation. Developed by Edmund Jacobson in the 1930s, it involves tightly contracting muscles, group by group, and then releasing the tension. This helps relax the body and also provides an effective way of learning how muscle tension feels in your body.

EMG biofeedback also produces muscle relaxation with the added trappings of modern technology. Meditation, as described in the last chapter, creates this same state of relaxation when used properly. In one study, progressive muscle relaxation improved the functioning of immune cells believed to defend the body against cancer in a group of elderly subjects.

What these techniques have in common is that they help create a state of relaxation. This facilitates a physiology of love, rather than fear, in our bodies and helps the healing process. Anything which balances our lifestyle will also help accomplish this. The Cayce readings encourage setting aside time for recreation and play to enjoy life. Time outdoors and in the sunshine is essential. The readings also encourage moderate exercise for all but the very ill. The need for maintaining a creative approach to life is often emphasized. Each of these suggestions will help create and maintain a physiology of love and grace in our bodies. Each will help us to live with the tapes we already have as we go through the more permanent process of changing them through meditation and working with our ideal.

6

Caring for Vital Circuits: The Role of the Spine

Osteopathy is one of the great revolutionizing ideas that light the course of history and mark its turning points. Other such great ideas have been the concepts of evolution and natural selection; quantum theory and the theory of relativity. The impact of osteopathy . . . will eventually be equally transforming.

I. M. KORR, PH.D.

There is no form of physical mechanotherapy so near in accord with nature's *measures as correctly given osteopathic adjustments.*

EDGAR CAYCE reading no. 1158–31

IT IS RARE TO find someone like Dr. Korr who speaks of osteopathy in the same glowing terms as the Cayce readings, at least one who can give you a reason for their praise. Dr. Korr spent most of his professional life researching why osteopathy works. He obviously was convinced of its value. Cayce certainly was convinced; the readings recommend osteopathic treatments in six thousand of the physical readings—about two-thirds of the total. When an individual asked what therapy could be used in lieu of osteopathic adjustments, the response came, "If there has been one found we haven't it yet!" (no. 1842–3). The readings go on to present a rationale for the recommended manipulations, a rationale substantiated by the existing research.

At the center of this therapeutic approach is the nervous system—the 10 billion neurons that act as the communication network to coordinate all of the body's activities. Each of these 10 billion neurons receives and sends messages with tens of thousands of others. In addition, each neuron is surrounded by an average of ten support cells called neuroglia, which research indicates are critical to the workings and even the survival of the neurons.

Maintaining a balance between the different parts of the nervous system is central to its health. When the system is out of kilter, the resulting impulses to various organs can cause chaos instead of order, disharmony instead of coordination. The Cayce readings link many diseases with just such a situation.

Bolstering the readings' position is experimental evidence that neurons which reach the various organs have very real effects on them. Nerve input serves to modulate the activity of each organ—causing it to quicken or slow. Medicine makes use of this. Drugs are used to block the nervous system's signals to the heart in order to slow it down or speed it up. Similarly, surgeons often cut the vagus nerve to reduce the amount of acid produced by the stomach.

In addition to directly innervating the organs, nerves play another major role in organ function—they control their blood supply. Every artery and vein is wrapped by nerve fibers which can change the vessel's diameter and affect how much blood flows through it. This blood supply is critical to the health of any portion of our body. The better the blood supply, the quicker the healing and the less risk of problems, regardless of the condition.

In addition to serving as a communication network with the organs and the blood vessels, the nervous system plays an even more basic role. Nerves have a trophic or nurturing function on the tissues they innervate. They are essential to the growth, development, self-maintenance, and survival of the cells they contact. Neurons have been shown to be critical in the process of determining what type of tissue a group of cells becomes as they develop.

With these capabilities, nerves can have dramatic effects on the healing process. In experiments done in the middle of the twentieth century, Russian scientist Alexander Speransky showed that cutting the nerves to various tissues can produce a large difference in the local inflammatory response. In one experiment, he injected hot tar into an animal's stomach lining. Normally, this produces a large cauliflower-like reaction. However, when he cut the vagus nerve, only a tiny lump would form. When he injected tuberculosis into the abdomen of an animal, it would rapidly spread throughout the animal's body. Once again, if the autonomic nerve supply to the abdomen was cut, there was very little tubercular spread, particularly to the lungs.

Speransky became convinced that the nervous system played a large role in the body's response to an infecting organism. During World War II, he treated Russian soldiers suffering from pneumonia with Novocain injections along the spine to alter existing nerve reflexes. Not all survived, but their rate of recovery was comparable to rates in the American army which used the new wonder, penicillin, and sulfa drugs. Speransky's astounding results invite others to confirm their accuracy by conducting similar experiments.

While science has apparently disregarded Speransky's work, scientists have conducted other studies that reveal similar dramatic results. One example involves asthma, a symptom complex in which the small air tubes in the lung constrict and make the passage of air very difficult. The result is the characteristic wheezing and shortness of breath. Studies have shown that by cutting the nerves to one lung, the problem in in that lung is relieved while the other lung, with nerves intact, will continue gasping for air.

A similar example involves the phenomenon of "shock lung," the flooding of the lungs with fluid after an injury to the brain. Working with Vietnam War casualties, doctors observed that fluid would never collect in the lungs if the head injury was accompanied by spinal injury. In other words, if the nerve connections between the injured brain and the lungs were severed, shock lung would not occur.

Surgeons and anesthesiologists sometimes accomplish a similar effect by removing or blocking the action of part of the sympathetic nervous system. Studies using these techniques have demonstrated accelerated wound healing and the altering of such symptoms as swelling, hives, redness, and itching. Studies with arthritics revealed relief of pain and increased mobility of the joints. Children with polio experienced restored bone growth on their affected side following interruption of the sympathetic nervous system. Even our sensory organs have been shown to be affected by the sympathetic nervous system, as increased stimulation can result in unnecessary firing of nerves with our brains receiving garbled, chaotic information.

Nerves carry power. They affect our body's cells structurally, functionally, and chemically. How can we influence this powerful regulatory system in our body? The Cayce readings believe skilled osteopathic manipulations are the answer.

This is not a new concept. Hippocrates recorded detailed suggestions for spinal traction and manipulation and Galen treated chariot drivers' cervical spines. In the early 1800s a group of "bonesetters" practiced widely in Europe. The idea took hold in the United States in the late nineteenth century with the work of a country doctor named Andrew Taylor Still. After the death of three of his children from spinal meningitis, Still became disillusioned with the medical approach of his day. He sought a new concept of healing and the field of osteopathy was born.

Currently, the term *manipulation* brings to mind chiropractors and their popping of vertebrae with high-velocity, low-amplitude thrust techniques. The Cayce readings describe osteopathic manipulations as being much more:

> Then the *science* of osteopathy is not merely the punching in a certain segment or the cracking of the bones, but it is the keeping of a *balance*—by the touch—between the sympathetic and the cerebrospinal system! *That* is real osteopathy! (no. 1158–24)

Manipulation, as a term, should mean any use of the hands to achieve maximal, painless movement of the musculoskeletal system to keep it in postural balance. This encompasses a full range of techniques from gentle ranging of a joint to the high velocity thrusts.

More than a snap, crackle, and pop, osteopathy involves extensive work with the soft tissue around the joints in an attempt to increase mobility. Soft-tissue work is considered by many osteopaths to be even more essential for complete healing than the more dramatic "clicking" and "popping" techniques.

Dr. Rex Conyers, an osteopath who studied the readings, interviewed fellow osteopaths who had been recommended in the readings. He found many who employed soft-tissue techniques almost exclusively in an attempt to mobilize each separate vertebra of the spine. One reported that the readings would occasionally tell him where to stand or sit while treating a patient. This practitioner noted that when he assumed these positions he was unable to apply any degree of force.

The Cayce readings also speak of very different effects that can be produced with the manipulative treatments.

> The osteopathic treatments are of these characters:
> There are those where stimulation of ganglia as related to the functioning of organs will assist in increasing the circulation to produce drainage.
> Or there may be such as to *prevent* drainage, or to prevent activity in this direction.
> And there are those where specific mechanical adjustments may be made. (no. 849–22)

This degree of specificity is becoming a lost art. There are, however, true masters still practicing in the United States and Europe who can do amazing things with the spine.

A key first step in working with spinal lesions is to make an accurate diagnosis. The therapeutic techniques chosen should be based on what is necessary to restore balance. Joints can be popped, whether beneficial or not, in any number of directions. Manipulation should be done with a purpose, and the ultimate purpose of any manipulation is to balance the nervous system and allow the body to self-regulate and move in the direction of health. The readings compare what a properly done osteopathic manipulation does for our body with what a piano tuner can do for a piano.

How can moving a joint bring the nervous system into balance? To answer this, we must understand what Dr. Korr called the "facilitated neuron." Dr. Korr's research demonstrated that nerves, under specific circumstances, require much less input from outside sources to fire than they normally would.

A number of things can cause a neuron to become hyperexcitable in the first place. Any condition which sends continuous signals to a neuron keeps it in a state of readiness. The readings indicate that facilitation can originate with problems in an organ, with the spine, or with the musculoskeltal system. If the colon, for example, is engorged and distressed, it may relay that message to the lumbar area and "facilitate" those nerves, causing spasm of the back muscles. The opposite may also occur. An injury to the back may cause lower back muscle spasm, facilitate the lumbar neurons, and eventually affect the colon. Finally, this same problem may start with an actual displacement (or subluxation) of the vertebral bodies.

The Cayce readings also imply that the places where nerves meet each other are important to maintain in optimal condition. They compare these connections with those of electrical wiring. Local "poisons" can create a form of corrosion at these sites, resulting in a short-circuiting of the nerve impulses.

Once a nerve becomes hyperexcitable, a variety of signals—many not intended for that particular neuron—can cause it to fire. Remember that each neuron connects with thousands of other neurons. The readings state that the connecting points between the central nervous system and the sympathetic nervous system act as special switches in this wiring system. As regulators of nerve impulses, these sites are especially affected by excess neuronal traffic. The end result is that nerve signals, which might normally just pass by, cause the facilitated neuron to fire.

To examine the implications of this, let's look at the case of an individual who is predisposed to asthmatic attacks. According to Dr. Korr's theory and the readings, the neuron which sends signals to the lung's air passageways to constrict—a normal function—is already poised to fire. Anything—nerve signals created by a response in the nose or mouth to pollen or an outpouring of nerve firings caused by an emotional event—has the potential to trigger that nerve to fire. And just a few such signals are necessary to keep the nerve firing fairly continuously. The result? The message gets conveyed to the lungs' airways, they constrict, and an asthmatic attack begins.

Give yourself a simple demonstration of the effects of a facilitated neuron. Lie on your back, lift your head, and place your fist (or some other small solid object) under your third cervical vertebrae. This can be found by first locating the inion—the bump in the center of your skull right above where your neck joins your head. Directly below this, find another large bump palpable in the soft tissue of your neck. This is your second cervical vertebrae. Directly below this would be your third cervical vertebrae.

Place your fist directly below this spot and rest your head on your hand for one to two minutes. Feel your sinuses and throat drain and clear. The readings say this simple technique "will drain, as it were, the whole system, setting up better eliminations . . ." (no. 3624–1).

By applying pressure to the neck, you increased the neuronal impulses arriving at that spinal segment. The result was an overflow of nerve impulses to other areas of your body, creating the drainage. Used for short intervals like this, such a technique can be helpful. However, any disruption of the normal equilibrium for any length of time will interfere with the balance of the system.

Excess and continuous stimulus to any organ will produce changes that will eventually manifest themselves as a dis-ease and then a disease. This may take 5 or 10 years to occur, but such constant bombardment eventually will take its toll. This concept might explain why, as we get older, certain parts of our bodies fail before the others do.

Each of us has our own pattern of "facilitation." It may not have reached the point of producing a complex of symptoms that we can identify as a disease. Nonetheless, it is there.

Dr. Korr conducted research in which he measured the temperature distribution on the skin's surface as a measure of sympathetic nervous system activity. He found two things. First, each of us has a unique pattern. Second, these patterns fall into identifiable groupings which he was able to connect with certain symptom complexes.

There was the stomach ulcer group, which was different from the duodenal ulcer group, both of which were different from the dysmenorrhea group, and so on. Often, the researchers would identify a certain pattern in an individual without symptoms. Over a period of time, however, especially if the individual was stressed, the predicted symptoms would appear.

There is a direct relationship between certain segments of our spine and our internal organs. The Cayce readings and science are in agreement about these relationships and they are presented below:

Heart T1–T4
Lungs and Airways T1–T6 } both of these are also supplied by the sympathetic nervous system from the cervical ganglia

Spleen T3–T10
Small Bowel T8–T11
Liver T8–T10
Colon
  -cecum and appendix T10–T12
  -transverse colon T12–L1
  -descending colon L1–L2
Stomach T6–T9 (T10 variable)
Gall Bladder T4–T9 (mainly T6–T9)
Pancreas T6–T9
Kidney T6–T12 (mainly T11–T12)
Bladder T11–L2
Uterus T11–L2

Key: T– thoracic or dorsal spine   L– lumbar spine
    Numbers refer to the vertebral level.

There are several ways we can identify and work with our particular pattern.

Traditionally, osteopaths have relied on an examination of the spine and the surrounding back muscles looking for asymmetry, hypo or hypermobility of joint range of motion, and changes in tissue texture. Let's address these one at a time.

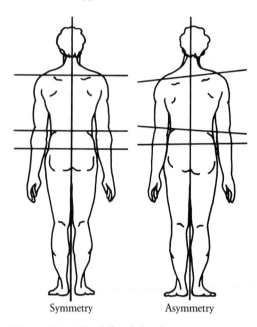

Symmetry   Asymmetry

Figure 6-1.   Check for skeletal symmetry.

Asymmetry of one side of our body as compared to the other side can be ascertained by observation and palpation. As a simple exercise, stand comfortably wearing few, if any, clothes and face a full-length mirror. Look closely at your body. Start by looking at your feet. Are they positioned evenly? Or does one turn out or in further than the other? Become aware of how you are bearing your weight. Does one leg bear more than the other? Is the distribution spread evenly along both feet from front to back and side to side? Next check the bony prominences of your hips, especially where they crest at your waist, as illustrated in Figure 6-1. Are they level?

Move to your shoulders and check their height. Now scan the soft tissue between your shoulders and your hips. Are the curves between your arms and your trunk the same shape and size on both sides? Is the muscle bulk of your chest (the pectoralis major muscle) and your shoulders (the trapezius muscle) equal on both sides? Are your neck and head perfectly vertical? A similar exam can be made by a friend or spouse of your back.

Now turn sideways. See if you can visually pass a straight line

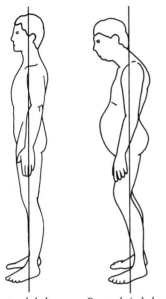

Postural balance   Postural imbalance

Figure 6-2. Check for postural balance.

from the front edge of your ear, through your shoulder tip, slightly behind the middle of your hip joint, and just along the front of your knee and ankle joints. Keeping these points aligned will maintain the vertebrae in optimal position, one on top of another, to produce the minimal strain on your spine. Figure 6-2 illustrates this principle of alignment.

The chances are excellent that you found some asymmetry. Does it mean anything? Sometimes it is clinically significant. Sometimes it is not. The next two steps in the diagnostic triad will help you to recognize which findings are significant. Treatment, however, will aim at building and maintaining more symmetry. Manipulation, therefore, should be accompanied by education regarding proper biomechanics and should be followed by an exercise program leading to postural balance. A good rule is to stretch where tight and strengthen where loose. The goal is the balance found in the middle-ground.

The other two diagnostic tools are more difficult to use in a self-exam. Changes in a joint's range of motion and the texture of surrounding tissue are the direct result of the hyperexcitability of the nerve supplying the area where the changes occur.

Acutely, the deep muscles of the back (especially the multifidus) go into spasm. You can create a similar muscle spasm by making a fist and holding it tightly for as long as you can. When doing this, your forearm muscles should be firm and tight—which is what a muscle in spasm feels like. Before long, you will feel some cramping and burning sensations and your arm may begin to tremble. With the muscle held tightly like this, blood cannot move through the muscle to deliver oxygen and to remove the waste products which are forming. As a result, acid builds up and produces the cramping, burning, and eventual pain.

With time, the blood vessels in the surrounding tissue dilate. Swelling and edema result and the tissue will feel boggy and doughy when touched. The skin may also feel slighter warmer than surrounding areas. This increased hydration will cause the skin to drag slightly when the finger tips are lightly run across the skin's surface. This feeling can be reproduced by taking a wristwatch off after an extended period of time. Moisture will have accumulated under the watch and will mimic the hydrated skin around an acute muscle spasm. Compare how your finger slides over the area which had been covered by the watch with the way it slides over the rest of your forearm.

The tissue edema will also affect the motion of adjacent joints. Instead of the free movement and smooth end-points you might normally find, the joint play will feel mushy and the end-points difficult to discern. The spasming muscle may also affect the directions in which the joint can move.

These same changes occur in the tissues adjacent to an acute spinal lesion. With practice, they can be palpated with your finger pads. Another test, which is easier but less specific, is skin rolling. To do this, move up and down the sides of the spine grabbing the skin between your thumb and your first two fingers. Roll it back and forth. The tissue adjacent to areas of altered function will be thickened, hardened, and tender.

These changes become self-perpetuating. The muscle spasm and the tissue changes irritate the local sensory nerves and signals are sent back to the spinal cord—further facilitating the involved neurons. Soft tissue work and mobilization of the joint decreases this flow of impulses to the beleagured neurons and allows them to rest and reequilibrate.

If a muscle continues to spasm, the feel of the tissue eventually changes. The blood vessels constrict and the swelling disappears. In its place, the tissue becomes fibrous and has a stringy feel. The temperature of the overlying skin may return to normal or become cooler than surrounding areas. The joint will again have an ease of motion, but with a greatly decreased range. Instead of reaching the end of this range smoothly, the joint motion will end early and abruptly.

These changes represent a chronic spinal lesion, in which decreased joint motion is established, making correction more difficult. They may also create patterns in the way our organs function—giving us our physiologic "weak spots." The goal of treatment at this point is to bring play back to the joint.

Treatment sessions should strive to impact, but not correct, the entire situation in one sitting—especially if chronic. Acute conditions can be treated frequently, up to daily, but with short sessions so as not to aggravate the situation. A chronic condition will tolerate longer sessions which can be spaced further apart—perhaps once a week. Overall, a given condition may respond in a single session or may take repeated treatments. A well-known osteopath, Dr. Phillip Greenman, has stated that if a condition has not responded in 12 weeks, it probably won't. After treatment is completed, the body can be reprogrammed with techniques from the Alexander, Feldenkrais, or PNF (proprioceptive neuromuscular facilitation) schools of thought to help maintain the new found balance.

A more subtle manifestation of spinal lesions may be revealed in what some researchers call our psychophysiological profile. Psychologists working with biofeedback have noticed that each of us has a unique pattern of response when our fight-or-flight mechanism is triggered by stress. Some of us show a great change in our heart rates. Others show greater change in skin conductance, while others have larger variations in blood pressure. Further research might indicate a relationship between these patterns and particular sets of "facilitated neurons." Such a relationship would be of great help clinically to the practitioner, as well as to us as individuals in our journey toward wholeness.

In addition to joint mobilization, two related techniques can also be helpful. The first is massage. The readings indicate that back and spine massage can indirectly help the nerve connections by improving the circulation around them. As a result, the supply of nutriments and the drainage of toxins is improved, preventing the "short-circuiting" of the nerve impulses.

The second technique involves applying pressure with a finger or the hands directly to the tender muscle or to an area reflexively related to it. This is similar to shiatsu, a Japanese technique sometimes called acupressure. Pressure will eventually fatigue the connecting nerve and the area will soon relax.

A more modern technique, using the same principle, is the use of Novocain injected into "trigger points." The injections deaden the nerve and stop the flow of impulses. Like an adjustment, this may give the facilitated neuron a chance to relax and rebalance.

These principles apply to each of us, regardless of age or health. Osteopathic lesions identify spinal segments and their related organs in which the probability of both dis-ease and disease is higher. We need to pay attention to these locations before they demand it from us in the form of organic problems.

7

Food for Thought: Eating for Health

And she had never forgotten that, if you drink much from a bottle marked "poison," it is almost certain to disagree with you, sooner or later.

LEWIS CARROLL, Alice in Wonderland

For without proper digestion all things look dark to any individual.

EDGAR CAYCE reading no. 288–9

Each one of us started this lifetime as a single cell. From the union of sperm and solitary egg emerged our current 70 trillion cells. The building blocks for each of these cells is obtained in only one way—assimilation into our bodies as food, water, or air.

Several hundred years ago alchemists were renowned for their claim of turning other metals into gold. Our bodies, after each meal, undergo a much less celebrated but equally astounding process. For "the blood supply is added to three times each day if meals are taken, else we would never recuperate or change a whole body every 7 years . . ." (no. 133–4). Plant and animal cells are converted into our own blood and bone and tissue. The butter on our bread becomes our cell membranes. The glucose in the orange we eat powers our brain and allows us to experience consciousness. As we nourish our cells, we improve our chances of thinking clearly, feeling vibrant, and being well.

There is ample evidence that lack of the right dietary tools can create massive problems for our bodies. In the late 1970s, a U.S. Senate Select Committee examined available studies and listened to testimony about our national eating habits. Their conclusion: diet is related to heart attacks, cancer, strokes, cirrhosis of the liver, arteriosclerosis, and diabetes—six of the ten leading causes of death in the United States. They found that diet not only can harm, it also can help. Nutritional and dietary factors have been shown conclusively to extend life expectancy of laboratory animals and decrease the rate, frequency, and severity of the six disorders listed above. The Senate report concluded:

> We have reached the point where nutrition . . . may be the nation's number-one public health problem. The threat is . . . millions of Americans loading their stomachs with food which is likely to make them obese, to give them high blood pressure, to induce heart disease, diabetes, and cancer—in short, to kill them over the long term.

The Cayce readings put it this way—"What we think and what we eat—combined together—make what we are, physically and mentally" (no. 288–38). That makes logical sense, yet most of us pay little attention to what we put in our systems. In 1981 the Pillsbury Company surveyed the eating habits of twenty thousand people. The results indicated that only 2 percent of these folks were "smart eaters," consuming adequate nutrients and calories.

Our apparent collective disinterest in an optimal diet is probably rooted in a number of complex issues. Culturally, we use food to insulate us from our emotions, relieve our pain, and serve as our security system. Additionally, nutrition is a highly charged subject on which the "experts" often have diametrically opposing viewpoints.

Such confusion has caused most of us to relinquish control over our eating habits. Rather than being in touch with our body's needs and choosing foods from a place of awareness and with a sense of self-responsibility, we follow patterns ingrained into us by our parents or the advertising media. As individuals who want to provide our bodies with the best building blocks, we face a real challenge.

The Cayce readings suggest that each of us make decisions about our diet based on "common good judgement, according to that which agrees and disagrees with the body" (no. 140–12). Implicit in this advice is the fact that the right diet for your body should make you feel better and over time you should be healthier as a result.

Also implied here is that what may be good for someone else may not be the best for you. As Lucretius said over two thousand years ago, "What is food to one man may be fierce poison to another." Biochemist-nutritionist Roger J. Williams observed, "If normal facial features varied as much as gastric juices do, some of our noses would be about the size of navy beans while others would be the size of 20-pound watermelons." Because of this, what works for one person may be the downfall of another. The Cayce material states there is "the necessity of watching, experimenting as it were with that which is good today and may be bad tomorrow. For what would be poison for someone, to another may be a cure" (no. 1259–2).

Despite individual differences, there are some guidelines which seem to apply to all of us. The Senate Select Committee, two hundred scientists from twenty-three countries reporting in the *Journal of the American Medical Association*, the *Surgeon General's Report on Nutrition and Health* published in 1988, and the Edgar Cayce readings agree on basic changes we all need to make in our diets. These include:

- Fewer total calories.
- Less fat.
- More grains, nuts, fruits, and vegetables.
- Less intake of processed foods.
- Less sugar.
- More fiber.

Following through on these recommendations would require most of us to change the ratio of calories we obtain from fats, carbohydrates, and proteins. Figure 7-1 illustrates the ratios of the typical American's diet. Part (b) shows the percentages recommended by the Senate committee. Part (c) is my estimate of the ratios suggested by the Cayce readings. As you see, suggestions from the readings recommend the same changes that emerged from the testimony of the nation's best nutritionists, only carried further.

The average American diet, as the diagram shows, is in many ways the opposite of the diet recommended by the Cayce readings, resulting from 50 years of continued veering away from the Cayce diet suggestions. Compared with the early 1900s, we are eating 50 percent more refined sugar, 33 percent more fat, and almost 50 percent less grains, fruits, and vegetables. While we are eating roughly the same amount of protein, we're getting much more of it now from meat and other fat-rich sources.

Should we change this trend? Nutritional experts, pointing to research on the effects of fats, proteins, and carbohydrates on the body, answer with a resounding yes.

Diets high in fat have been directly linked with heart disease and cancer and indirectly with hypertension, gall bladder disease, diabetes, and liver disease. There is also a connection between dietary fat and degenerative diseases. Societies with less than 20 percent of their calories coming from fat have a low incidence of these diseases.

Fat seems to adversely affect the body in several ways. First, it causes the blood to thicken, resulting in sludging and blockage of capillaries. This decreases the oxygen available to the body's cells.

Second, fat affects the gut by altering the balance of bacteria and producing up to ten times the normal amount of bile acids. Anaerobic bacteria, those that don't need oxygen, increase and can convert the increased bile acids into carcinogens.

Third, dietary fat increases the cholesterol level in the blood. Cholesterol is like a wax and does not dissolve easily in the blood plasma. There is now *lots* of evidence that a person's cholesterol level is directly related to their risk of coronary heart disease. In numerous studies, scientists have found that they can cause *and* reverse arterial plaque disease by altering the amount of dietary fat and cholesterol.

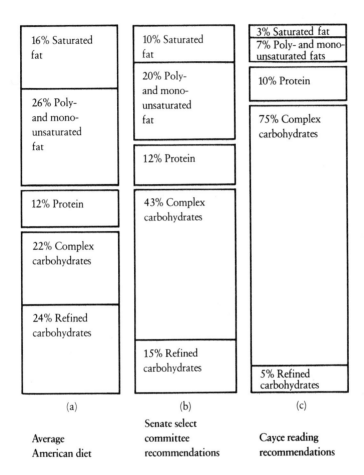

Figure 7-1. **Dietary ratios of fats, proteins, and carbohydrates.**

Finally, studies have demonstrated that raised blood levels of free fatty acids produce higher blood sugar levels and decrease the response of cells to insulin. This may play a role in the disease of diabetes mellitus.

How much fat do we need in our diets? No one knows for sure, but it is certainly far less than we currently consume. The only fat the body cannot make on its own is linoleic acid and our daily requirement of this is so small that an ounce of oatmeal will satisfy it. The average American diet has 42 percent of the calories consumed as fat. Yet, one study published in the American Journal of Clinical Nutrition in 1970 put adult males on a diet consisting of only 0.7 percent fat for six months without them developing any adverse symptoms.

Such drastic reductions probably are unrealistic. Fat helps give texture and taste to our food. It also helps us feel full for longer periods of time by slowing down the process of food leaving our stomachs. Additionally, certain essential vitamins are ingested with fats. A balance needs to be obtained. The Cayce readings sometimes suggest that individuals take a tablespoon of olive oil, describing it as a "food" for the intestines. But the readings also warned against cooking with grease and eating fatty red meats.

Our protein intake also needs to be examined. Americans' protein consumption is roughly twice the recommended daily allowance for most healthy people. This extra protein is a burden to the body's elimination systems, and some of its breakdown products, like ammonia, can be very toxic to the body. Meat also contains phosphorus, which in large amounts sends us into a negative mineral balance, especially affecting calcium levels. Furthermore, meat is often the vehicle for much of the fat we eat.

While Americans' protein intake has remained at approximately 12 percent since the turn of the century, the ratio of animal to vegetable protein has doubled. Even before this change, the readings were encouraging people to eat meat in moderation. The majority of protein in our diets should come from vegetable sources. The meat that is consumed should consist mainly of fish, fowl, and lamb. Red meat should be consumed once a week or less. The calories in steak are divided roughly between protein and fat. In contrast, fish and chicken have a ratio of 75 percent or more protein to 25 percent or less fat. For unspecified reasons, the readings express a preference for wild game when it is available.

Pork, with the exception of occasional crisp bacon for breakfast, is never to be eaten, according to the readings. They go on to indicate that pork and ham are very difficult to digest and leave by-products in the body which are hard to eliminate and can collect in the tissue as crystals.

Based on the foregoing information, it's logical to ask whether meat is necessary at all. Here the readings defer to individual differences. Several people were told in readings that their body required meat. Others were told to stop eating meat for spiritual reasons, though one individual was told to "spiritualize those influences . . . rather than abstaining" (no. 295–10). Most often the choice was left to the individual. To those who chose not to eat meat, the readings sometimes recommended "supplements, either in vitamins or in [meat] substitutes" (no. 5401–1). Overall, however, when compared to the amount of meat we consume today, the Cayce regimen can be viewed as being semivegetarian.

The final way we obtain the calories necessary to drive our system is carbohydrates. These come in a variety of forms, but can be broken into two major categories—those which are complex or "natural" and those which are refined. The latter group is responsible for the bad press that carbohydrates have received in the past several years.

Sugar, being highly refined, lacks vitamins, minerals, and fiber. Essentially, it is a source of empty calories. Currently the average American obtains twenty-five percent of dietary calories from sugar, which averages out to every man, woman, and child eating one-third of a pound of sugar a day. (Three-fourths of this comes in the form of processed foods.) That means that the other 75 percent of our caloric intake must supply 100 percent of the nutrients our bodies require. Additionally, refined sugars need no digestion; they flood the system and then quickly disappear, sending our bodies on hormonal roller-coaster rides. Refined sugars also contribute to atherosclerosis by raising the blood levels of fats and cholesterol.

Carbohydrates do, however, come in many other forms—including fruits, vegetables, and grains. In the early 1900s, these three foods comprised 40 percent of peoples' diets. Today we get less than 20 percent of our calories from these sources. The Cayce readings, over and over again, clearly state that people in Cayce's time should have eaten more fruits and a lot more vegetables than they did. The readings indicate that fruits and vegetables should comprise between 60 and 80 percent of the diet!

There is good sense in this. Unlike sugar, complex carbohydrates require digestion and enter the bloodstream at a slow and steady rate—keeping the fires of metabolism burning at a constant level. And unlike fats and proteins, carbohydrates burn 100 percent clean—the only breakdown products being water and carbon dioxide.

The Cayce readings often refer to fruits and vegetables as body-building foods and have high praise for them. The readings say that certain vegetables, especially lettuce, are blood purifiers which would help the body resist any type of infection. Others, like raw celery and carrots, play a special role in nourishing the nerves.

Whether these benefits are the result of the ample supply of vitamins and minerals in vegetables is not made clear by the readings. They do, however, make some recommendations regarding vitamins which are worth noting. Consistent with their approach to the body, the readings strike a note of balance in their view on vitamins. On the one hand, the readings tout vitamins as "The creative forces working with the body-energies for the renewing of the body!" (no. 3511–1). In this role, they are stated to be "food for the glands," supplying the "energies to enable the varied organs of the body to reproduce themselves" (no. 2072–9). On the other hand, the readings seem to anticipate their commercialization and exploitation, stating that each vitamin was a "combination of . . . other influences—given a name mostly for confusion . . . by those who would tell you what to do for a price!" (no. 2533–6).

The readings' attitude towards vitamins might be summed up with the statement "nature still does it best." Whenever possible, vitamins are to be obtained in the quantities and ratios found in wholesome foods, especially vegetables. Gelatin is recommended to be consumed with salads to help with the assimilation of the vitamins.

While megadose vitamin therapies are never recommended, supplements (especially of the B vitamins) are often suggested. These are to be used for short intervals, when the body is run down for any reason—stress, illness, or debilitation—or when the diet is not being kept at the level it should be—as in the winter when quality fresh produce may not be available. When supplements are used, they are to be taken in cycles so that the body will not lose its pattern of absorbing them from the regular diet and become dependent on the supplements for its supply. Pills are never to take the place of eating good quality foods.

In addition to vitamins and minerals, complex carbohydrates also provide the fiber we need in our diets. Two British physicians, Dennis Burkitt and Hugh Trowell, conducted studies of different African peoples after noting that they had a negligible incidence of coronary heart disease, colon cancer, diverticulosis, varicose veins, gallbladder disease, and constipation. They found that these people also had a large amount of fiber in their diets. Fiber gives bulk to the stool which helps move it through the gut and, in the process, removes toxins and carcinogens from the body more quickly.

So, there are ample reasons for changing the ratio of the food types we consume. As we have noted, the readings' suggestions agree with the current thinking of the American Cancer Society, the American Heart Association, the Senate's Select Committee, and other organizations. However, as they often do, the Cayce readings go beyond these insights and provide another reason which is rarely discussed and is controversial. This involves the maintenance of an "acid-alkaline balance" in the body.

Cayce was asked by one individual to give general rules to obtain and maintain better health. The response urged care in keeping a proper balance in the person's acid-alkaline state. Our bodies work hard to maintain and live at a slightly alkaline pH of 7.4. (The pH scale goes from 1 to 14, with 7.0 being neutral. Anything below 7.0 represents an acidic condition, anything above 7.0 represents an alkaline state.) This involves maintaining a certain electronic balance of ions or charged particles in the bloodstream. Foods can affect this with the positive or negative charges which remain after they have been digested and metabolized at the cellular level. The readings stressed that one way to help the body stay balanced is to consume a ratio of 80 percent alkaline-producing foods to 20 percent acid-producing foods.

Alkaline-producing foods include most fruits and vegetables. Their digestion leaves an ash in which the majority of elements are positively charged—potassium, sodium, calcium, and magnesium. Cereals and meats leave an ash which has a greater number of negatively charged ions—such as chlorine, phosphorus, iodine, and sulfur—and this residue has an acid-producing effect on the body. Below are lists that outline which foods fit into these two categories.

Alkaline-Forming Foods—Eighty percent, or four-fifths, of one's diet should come from these foods:

- All vegetables except for lentils and corn.
- All fruits, fresh and dried, except for cranberries, plums, and prunes.
- All forms of milk.
- Almonds, chestnuts, Brazil nuts, and hazelnuts.

Acid-Forming Foods—Twenty percent, or one-fifth, of one's diet should come from these foods:

- All meats except for mincemeat.
- All cereals and bakery products except for soybeans.
- Cheese and eggs.
- Peanuts, pecans, and walnuts.

These foods probably do not affect the actual pH of the blood. The body has numerous buffer systems to help keep it stabilized right around 7.4, as this is critical to life. However, these foods do affect the body's buffer systems and, in the process, affect the red blood cells, the kidneys, and other cells in the body.

The readings suggest that the easiest way to monitor the status of the system is through watching the pH of the urine or saliva, as these will change as the diet is changed. For our purposes, monitoring the saliva is probably the simplest. Saliva normally has a pH range of 6.0 (acidic) to 7.9 (alkaline). The best way to monitor one's own saliva is with the use of blue litmus paper. To do this, take a single paper strip and wet it with saliva. If the paper stays blue, then the pH is 7.0 or above and the body is in an alkaline state. If the paper turns pink, the pH of the saliva is below 7.0, indicating that the body is an acid state.

The best time to test the saliva is on awakening in the morning as meals can affect the saliva's pH for up to 5 or 6 hours. The readings suggest that we monitor our body in this way about once a week. If the body is found to be in an acid state, with the saliva turning the blue litmus paper pink, the readings suggest consuming citrus fruits at that morning meal to help the body rebalance.

In general, the more physically active a person is, the more acid-producing foods they can have in their diet because "*energies* or activities . . . burn acids, but those who lead the sedentary life or the non-active life can't go on sweets or too much starches . . ." (no. 798–1). The readings also say that a person, when ill, needs to reduce the amount of acid-producing foods they consume for there is "the natural inclinations of disturbed conditions in a body . . . to produce acidity through the blood stream" (no. 1302–1). The tendency, then, should be toward a slightly alkaline state. However, if one is to err, it is more detrimental to become too alkaline than it is to be too acidic.

In addition to the concept of an acid-alkaline balance, the readings make other dietary suggestions which are not commonly heard. These cover such areas as food combining, acclimatization, attitude during eating, and consuming foods in harmony with the body cycles.

Let's start by looking at attitude. We know that one-third of the body's neurons are in the gut. We also know that the autonomic nervous system richly innervates and communicates with those neurons, making the bowel very reactive to our emotional states. Because of this, the readings strongly emphasize that one should "never [when] under strain, when very tired, very excited, very mad, . . . take foods [into] the system" (no. 137–30).

One should also "take *time* to eat and to eat the right thing" (no. 243–23). Such awareness should begin before the meal. Many cultures and religions share the tradition of a prayer before eating. This time can serve as a few moments to rest, to bless both the food and one's body, and to visualize the food helping the body.

This awareness should then carry over to actual eating practices.

The readings make clear that chewing is the first step in the digestive process and is important in the assimilation process. They agree with Walt Whitman's admonition to "Drink your solids and chew your liquids." In fact, the readings indicate that "bolting food or swallowing it by the use of liquids produces more colds than *any one* activity of a diet" (no. 808–3).

Finally, awareness needs to extend past the meal, recognizing that our bodies undergo a major shift in blood flow to help the digestive process. As a result, it is helpful to have a period of rest after meals, especially lunch, "before becoming so mentally and bodily active as to upset digestion" (no. 243–23).

Another helpful concept found in the readings is that certain combinations of food types help or hinder the intestinal system. One individual asked Cayce what foods should be avoided. The response was that no particular food needs to be avoided, "rather is it the combination of foods that makes for disturbances with most physical bodies" (no. 416–9). As an example, grains and citrus fruit are repeatedly recommended as good foods. However, the warning was frequently given that these two should not to be taken together. "For this *changes* the acidity in the stomach to a detrimental condition; for citrus fruits will act as an eliminant when taken alone, but when taken with cereals it becomes as weight. . ." (no. 481—1). Food combinations, recommended and warned about in the readings, are given below.

Food Combining

These are foods recommended to be eaten together:

- Gelatin and salad to help with nutrient absorption.
- Small amounts of lemon or lime juice with orange or grapefruit juice.
- At least three vegetables that grow above the ground for each one that grows under the ground.
- Figs, dates, and cornmeal as a cleanser and "spiritual food."

These are foods to avoid eating together:

- Two or more starchy foods at the same meal.
- Sugary foods and starchy foods.
- Milk and citrus fruit or juice.
- Citrus fruit or juice and cereals.
- Starchy foods with meat or cheese.
- Coffee with milk or cream.
- Raw apples with other foods.

These food-combining principles do eliminate many American dietary favorites, like macaroni and cheese, and meat and potatoes. There are, however, *many* foods to take their place. To balance the diet, do not combine foods, but rotate them.

Food-combining principles can be understood with what we know about the physiology of the digestive system. These ideas were first outlined in 1902 by Ivan Pavlov in *The Work of the Digestive Glands*. The basic concept of these principles comes from the fact that proteins, like meat, require one set of conditions for their digestion, while starches require another. The enzymes to digest protein work best in an acidic environment; the enzymes to digest starches require the pH to be above seven. The two are just not compatible.

Acclimatization, or the eating of locally grown foods, is another dietary concept found in the Cayce readings. There are at least two reasons why locally grown foods are better for us. First, the fresher the produce is, the better. Vegetables lose their vitamin content fairly quickly. The second reason is that when we eat local food, "this prepares the system to acclimate itself to any given territory" (no. 3542–1)—helping the body to adjust to the weather and other environmental conditions.

The Cayce readings also offer ideas on when certain foods should be eaten relative to body cycles. The general concept is that nerve-building foods should be eaten at breakfast and lunch, and blood-building foods consumed at dinner. This translates into cereals or citrus fruit for breakfast. Lunch is the ideal meal for uncooked foods like salad or raw vegetables. Meats and cooked vegetables are reserved for the evening meal. A typical day's menu looks like this:

Breakfast
Either citrus fruit, *or* cooked or dry cereal with milk.

Lunch
Raw vegetable salad with dressing *or* fruit salad.

Dinner
Cooked vegetables served with fish, poultry, or lamb.

Finally, the Cayce readings have some ideas about food preparation. The first and foremost of these is a constant warning about frying food. "Never anything fried" are familiar words to anyone who has studied the readings. The frying process, according to the readings, changes food in such a way that it disturbs the functioning of the liver and gall bladder.

On the positive side, the readings recommend that vegetables be cooked in Patapar Paper, a specially processed parchment that keeps the vegetable juices concentrated and helps preserve their vitamins. The vegetables are tied in the paper and immersed in boiling water.

These concepts form the beginning guidelines from which each of us can experiment and learn what works best for our body. In working with these principles, eating should remain a joy and never become an obsession. In the words of the readings, "Then the diet: this should not be so rigid . . . but rather . . . let . . . every activity [be] purposeful in conception, constructive in nature" (no. 1183–2).

8

Inner Pollution Solutions: Maintaining Eliminations

For the system . . . is able to bring resuscitation so long as the eliminations do not hinder.
EDGAR CAYCE reading no. 311–4

My people are destroyed for lack of knowledge.
HOSEA 4:6

HAVE YOU EVER FELT sluggish? An achy, dragging feeling of heaviness and fatigue can occur when the systems that process your body's wastes aren't keeping up. When your body is in another cycle, these wastes may have the opposite effect and you may feel restless and nervous. Or the condition may manifest itself as a headache or skin condition. Some scientists go so far as to suggest that aging can be explained by the accumulation over time of the toxic by-products of our body's metabolism.

We are not only what we eat and think, but we also are what we don't get rid of. This does not require a vivid imagination. Any environment is most desirable and healthy to live in when it is clean.

We have many sources of waste material, but four are particularly worth mentioning. First there are the byproducts of normal metabolism. Every cell in its normal functioning produces what the readings call ash or drosses. Many of these are toxic to the body. As an example, virtually all of our cells produce ammonia as they break down the building blocks of protein—the amino acids. Nitrogen, in this form, can cause blurred vision, tremors, slurred speech, and—in extreme cases—cause even coma and death. Very simply, this waste needs to be processed and removed.

In this same category are the free radicals. These are atoms or molecules which have an unpaired electron and therefore are very reactive. These free radicals are both essential to many life processes and at the same time highly destructive if not contained by the body's natural control mechanisms. They may be responsible for many of our ailments, from arthritis and atherosclerosis to diabetes, and for the process of aging.

A second and related source of material which needs to be handled by the body are the 300 to 800 billion cells which die daily in our bodies as part of the natural process of regeneration. Each of these cells contain residual bodies of wastes they couldn't digest or expel. They also contain unused pockets of powerful digestive enzymes known as lysosomes. Normally contained by a protective membrane, these enzymes are released into the surrounding tissue when a cell dies. The readings compare the poisons generated from destroyed cells to "grains of sand" and state that they can affect the blood's circulation like "rust in a pipe."

The third and fourth sources of unwanted substances come from outside the body. Our diet can introduce waste directly into our systems and can also contribute to an intestinal environment in which eliminations are hindered and further toxins are produced. In addition, our bodies are now constantly deluged with ever more complex and dangerous molecules in the form of thousands of food additives and environmental pollutants.

Fortunately, the body comes equipped with four separate waste disposal systems: (1) the skin and sweat glands, (2) the lungs, (3) the kidneys, and (4) the liver and digestive tract. Each is exquisitely constructed and highly capable of its task. In fact, all work so well that traditional medicine has had difficulty accepting the idea that the average person is adversely affected by their own waste. The liver and the kidneys, for example, can suffer up to 75 percent destruction before impairment of their functioning is evident. The skin covers an average of 17 square feet, containing about two million sweat glands. The lungs have approximately 300 million alveoli which if flattened out would cover half a tennis court.

It is rare, therefore, to see the dramatic symptoms of total organ failure: the thirst, nausea and vomiting, itching, and sallow complexion of a person whose kidneys have shut down. Or the swollen body, bluish color, and labored breathing of the individual whose lung passages have been obstructed from years of smoking. Or the jaundice, bloated abdomen, and mental confusion of the chronic alchoholic in liver failure.

And yet the Cayce readings, in case after case, make clear that proper eliminations are one of the basic keys to our health. Rather than organ failure, they focus on two other possible disturbances. First, the readings make clear that each of the elimination systems has an optimal level of activity. Disturbances of blood supply or nerve input can overstimulate or produce a sluggish response. This, in turn, can affect the second area—subtle disturbances of the delicate interplay between these organs. Many readings emphasize that the first step in working with many diseases is to optimize the functioning of these elimination systems to help the body eradicate the problem.

One relationship the readings repeatedly stress is the delicate balance between the liver and the kidneys. According to the readings, numerous health problems have their origin in the breakdown of this relationship. It is mentioned as important in such diverse situations as tuberculosis, diabetes, rheumatism, acne, eye and ear problems, and naturally, liver and kidney diseases.

Both the liver and the kidneys are complex and vital organs. The liver is referred to as the chemical factory of the body with more than five hundred important metabolic functions attributed to it. When the body is at rest, one-quarter of its blood is within the liver being processed. The kidneys completely process the body's blood three to four hundred times every 24 hours—a total of approximately 1,800 liters in a day.

The relationship between the liver and kidneys seems to correspond to the electrical nature of the body. The readings speak of the body as a battery with the liver and the kidneys as its poles—one the positive, the other negative. Any disturbance between these poles produces a short-circuit in their functioning, causing poisons that should be eliminated to be thrown back into the system.

One way this relationship manifests itself is that the two organs pick up the slack for each other. As the activity of one decreases, the other's activity increases. In the majority of readings, this involves a congested or torpid liver and overworked kidneys. One effect of this condition is to alter the circulation pattern of the blood in the abdomen.

This concept has found support in research and clinical experience. The most dramatic example is the kidney failure which can occur in patients with cirrhosis, known as hepatorenal syndrome. With rare exceptions, it is fatal and is one of the primary ways persons with cirrhosis die. Amazingly, however, the kidneys in these individuals are still capable of operating normally and have worked well after being transplanted to another person. There is nothing actually wrong with them. The reason they shut down is that their blood supply is greatly decreased. The Cayce readings indicate that this process is constantly occuring in a subtle fashion in all of us.

Many of the recommendations in this book are directed at maintaining an optimal balance between the different systems of elimination, especially the liver and kidneys.

Many of these suggestions make use of the natural cleansing properties of water. Water and life are synonymous; the body will not survive without water. In addition to being needed for the eliminations, it also cools the body, is vital to the process of digestion, and becomes the medium which transports needed nutrients to every cell. So, it comes as no surprise that water has been used in healing for thousands of years—baths and other water remedies appear in Sanskrit records as early as 4000 B.C. Water has been used symbolically in many civilizations to cleanse, sanctify, and purify.

Water *is* critical to all four elimination systems—even the skin. We can lose up to 6 cups of water in a day through our skin without any obvious perspiration, and each drop contains lactic acid and urea—both toxic to the body.

The simplest use of water in healing is the mere act of drinking it. The Cayce readings told many individuals that they should consume between 6 and 8 glasses of water a day. That is much harder than it sounds, but it is vital to our well-being. Everything needs washing to stay clean—we shower and wash our clothes regularly. Similarly, each of the 70 trillion cells in our bodies benefits from being washed with a daily 6 to 8 glasses of water. The liver, the gut, and kidneys especially benefit from the intake of water. With these working properly, the lungs and skin are not overtaxed.

A side benefit of water is the help it provides to the stomach. The readings indicate that as food is consumed, the stomach, immediately "becomes a storehouse, or a medicine chest that may create all the elements necessary for proper digestion within the system" (no. 311–4). Water helps the stomach function at its optimum by keeping it slightly dilated. In particular, half a glass of warm water on first awakening was recommended as a way to help the digestive system work best.

Another function for water recommended time and again by the readings is in colonics. "For *every* one—everybody—should take an internal bath occasionally as well as an external one. They would all be better off if they would" (no. 440–2). It does not take a vivid imagination to extrapolate to our colon from the analogy of what happens to our bodies when we don't shower. While no research has been attempted to validate the importance of colonics, such cleansing makes common sense.

For a colonic, a teaspoon to a tablespoon each of salt and sodium bicarbonate should be mixed with each gallon of rinse water so there is no adverse effect on the colon's electrolyte or pH balance. The final rinse waters should contain a tablespoon of Glyco-Thymoline to a gallon of water, serving as an intestinal antiseptic to purify the system. For a variety of reasons, colonics should be professionally administered by an experienced individual. Unfortunately, such colonic services are not always readily available, but a home enema is. While a colonic has the effect of four to six enemas, any internal bath is better than none.

An enema can be self-administered easily at home using one of the bag setups available commercially. Start by sterilizing the nozzle or tube before using it. Then, mix a teaspoon of salt and sodium bicarbonate in a quart of lukewarm (98.6 ° F) water. Begin by lying on your left side with towels and/or plastic material placed beneath you to protect the bed or the rug. Coat the enema tube with vaseline and insert it 2 to 4 inches into your rectum. (CAUTION: Do not force it.) Allow one-third of the water into your rectum, controlling the water speed to prevent cramping. If you feel you cannot hold the water, clamp the tube and take a few deep breaths before continuing. After a third of a quart is in, turn and lie on your back without removing the nozzle. Allow another third of a quart in using the same process. Then turn on your right side and allow the final third to pass into your colon. Your colon circles your abdomen as shown in Figure 8-1, and this maneuvering is to get the enema solution around its corners.

Once the solution is in, try to retain the water for 5 to 15 minutes before expelling it, moving to swish it around. After finishing, rest for several minutes, and then repeat this process until the expelled fluid is largely clear and without solid material. The final enema should contain a teaspoonful of Glyco-Thymoline (instead of salt and soda) in a quart of water.

Another role for water is in special baths. Two particularly recommended are Epsom-salt baths and fume or sweat baths. The Epsom salts are useful in helping with eliminations through the skin and are recommended for such varied conditions as lower back pain, nerve inflammation, arthritis and other joint pain, and for liver and kidney imbalance and sluggishness.

An Epsom-salt bath is easy to take at home. In general, use about 5 pounds for a regular tub (about 20 gallons of water) and 8 to 10 pounds for a larger whirlpool or old-fashioned tub. Stir the salts thoroughly so that they dissolve well. Begin with the water temperature at 102 to 104° F—use a thermometer to check this. Gradually

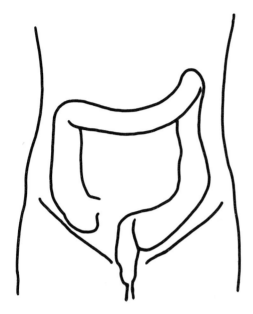

Figure 8-1. The large intestine.

add hot water and progressively raise the temperature to 106 to 112° F. Make sure the affected areas get in the water and are well soaked. Stay in the water 10 to 12 minutes initially, and as your body acclimates to the heat over several baths, gradually increase this time to 20 minutes. The readings often recommended a massage—either general or to the affected area—during the bath or immediately following it.

It is helpful to have someone nearby in case you feel dizzy or faint and to keep track of the time for you. A cool washcloth on the forehead or back of the neck will help you tolerate the heat. When finished, shower to wash off the salt. (CAUTION: Hot baths of any kind are not recommended if you have heart disease, high blood pressure, have any chance of being pregnant, or are coming off steroid therapy. In such cases, consider using an Epsom-salt pack applied to the affected area only. This can be made by thoroughly saturating a coarse cotton or linen cloth that has a loose weave with Epsom salts dissolved in water. Apply to the desired area and cover with a dry towel and leave until cool.)

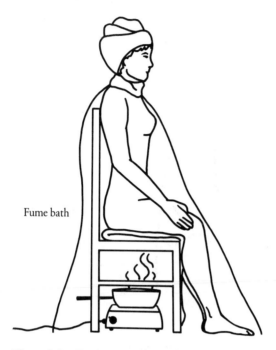

Fume bath

Figure 8-2. Do-it-yourself home fume bath.

Another technique to help with eliminations are fume baths. These also have additional benefits. The readings often encouraged their use to strengthen the body and aid the process of rejuvenation by adding such substances as witch hazel, Atomidine, lavender oil, myrrh, eucalyptus oil, or pine needle oil to the simmering water. While these baths are a bit involved, they are possible to use in the home setting as well.

Place a hot plate and pot of boiling water (use one of the substances mentioned above, if desired) directly under a simple straight chair. Drape towels over the chair so that you don't risk burning your buttocks or legs. Drink 3 to 4 glasses of water, then sit undressed on the chair—draping a sheet, blanket, or fireproof plastic cover around your shoulders to create a tent to capture and hold the steam. Take another towel and wrap it around your neck to prevent the steam from escaping at the top of tent, as shown in Figure 8-2.

Start with a 5- to 10-minute session and gradually build up. A friend to assist you is helpful—being provided with drinking water (every 5 to 10 minutes) will keep you hydrated and allow for increased perspiration. In addition, your friend can check your pulse at the neck and monitor your oral temperature. Keep your pulse below 140 and the oral temperature under 104° F by regulating the amount of steam produced. End the fume bath with a cleansing shower. Like the Epsom-salt bath, fume baths should be followed with a thorough rubdown to help stimulate the circulation in the skin.

The four eliminating systems also can be aided and influenced with other techniques, in addition to use of water. Many of the dietary suggestions in Chapter Seven help directly or indirectly. More vegetables and fruit in the diet and the subsequent increase in fiber consumption are an example of this. Decreased fat intake, proper food combining, and the intake of alkaline-reacting foods also directly help the organs of elimination.

One technique that has been used through the ages, often with religious practices, is fasting. One of its major benefits appears to be the release of toxins stored in the body's fatty tissues. The readings say total fasting is more of a spiritual exercise than a health practice, and they often reminded the individual that true fasting is casting out of self—"laying aside thine own concept of *how* or *what* should be done at this period, and [letting] the *Spirit* guide" (no. 295–6). For the purposes of cleansing the physical body, the readings recommend two diet techniques as being superior to a total fast.

The first is to follow the diet outlined in Chapter Seven. This assists the coordination of the entire system. The second method, as a way to directly release and eliminate toxins, is the use of certain special diets.

The most frequently recommended of these special diets is the apple diet. "This is to cleanse the activities of the liver, the kidneys, and the whole system" (no. 1850–3), and involves a mono-diet of Delicious or Jonathan apples—preferably organically grown so they are free of pesticides—and plenty of water for 3 days.

Eat five to six apples daily. On the evening of the third day, take from 1 tablespoon to half a cup (more frequently suggested) of olive oil. Castor oil packs (to be discussed later in the chapter) can be used before, but not during, the diet to stimulate the abdomen. "Three days of raw apples and then olive oil and we will cleanse all toxic forces from any system" (no. 820–2).

While this apple regimen is the most frequently mentioned special diet, the readings also recommended 4-day grape and 5-day citrus fruit mono-diets for cleansing. Follow these also with a dose of olive oil at the end.

Another special diet that occasionally is recommended to help eliminations and to better balance the alimentary canal is the combination of yogurt and fresh buttermilk. This can help with establishing the right bacteria in the intestines. Yogurt as part of one's regular diet is also suggested.

In addition to water and specific diets, there are other suggestions in the readings to help the elimination systems. These suggestions include teas and packs to stimulate the liver and the kidneys and eliminants to help the digestive tract.

Probably the best known of these techniques, and most deserving of special recognition, is the castor oil pack. Castor oil has been used since ancient times for a variety of medicinal purposes. The Romans referred to it as the *Palma Christi*, or hand of Christ. It is best known now as an evacuant of the alimentary canal when taken internally.

The Cayce readings recommend the castor oil pack almost exclusively to be used on the upper and lower right side of the abdomen. Its major physiological effect involves the stimulation of the liver, but it also stimulates the gall bladder and colon, which further assists eliminations. In the process, the readings say the pack improves the lymphatic circulation, dissolves adhesions, reduces inflammation, and improves assimilations in the intestines. Materials needed for a castor oil pack include cold-pressed castor oil and wool or cotton flannel (wool is preferred). A towel, plastic sheet, safety pins, and an electric heating pad also are helpful.

Soak the flannel with castor oil so that it is thoroughly saturated but not drippy (the oil can be prewarmed). Fold the flannel into two to four layers of thickness with the final size being determined by the area where it is to be applied. A standard pack applied to the abdomen is approximately 10 by 14 inches. The pack can be covered by the plastic sheet after it is placed on the skin. Place the heating pad over the plastic. The towel, the final layer, is wrapped around the body and held in place with safety pins to hold the ends together. Turn on the heating pad and heat the pack to your tolerance. (CAUTION: If a deep inflammatory process, like appendicitis, is suspected, the pack should not be heated.)

The readings most frequently suggest leaving the castor oil pack in place for 1 hour. Apply it in this way 3 days a week for 2 to 3 weeks. Then skip 1 week before resuming another cycle of treatment.

How do these packs work? The full answer is not yet known. One explanation from the readings for castor oil's effects is that it acts as a "limbering agent, or [allows] movement" (no. 1523–15)—similar to oil on a hinge. Harvey Grady, at the A.R.E. Clinic, in Phoenix, Arizona, has recently found some interesting studies in the scientific research literature that help explain why castor oil has a beneficial effect.

First, castor oil easily penetrates the skin. It does this so well, in fact, that studies have been done to examine its value as a vehicle to help get other medications into the body. Clearly castor oil affects more than just the skin.

Next, researchers have learned why castor oil is so successful in causing diarrhea when taken orally: the major active component of castor oil—ricinoleic acid—is converted by the body into a naturally occurring group of molecules known as prostaglandins. Prostaglandins, among the most potent biologic substances discovered to date, have hormonelike qualities and are involved in many important bodily functions. One of their best-known actions is to stimulate contractions of smooth muscle—the kind found in the abdomen.

Studies also have found that prostaglandins play an important role in protecting cells in the gut. They prevent the death of stomach cells following contact with acid, boiling water, and concentrated alcohol. Ulcers and other injuries to the small intestine, commonly seen with the use of certain medications, have been prevented. Finally, prostaglandins prevented an experimentally induced inflammation in the colon. In this experiment, castor oil was the most effective of the tested agents in producing this result.

Castor oil packs may also influence the immune system. Prosta-glandins are known to affect many of the different types of cells that are part of our bodies' defense system. In a recent study, the prosta-glandins most stimulated to production by castor oil were found to affect T-cell function and cell-mediated immunity in general.

More research is necessary, but this connection presents some exciting possibilities. Castor oil *does* affect how cells respond to the world around them. As the details of how it does this continue to be worked out, castor oil packs remain a valuable addition to anyone's home medicine kit.

As a counterbalance to the effect of the castor oil on the liver, the Cayce readings recommend the use of spirits of turpentine (CAU-TION: turpentine may burn the skin of some individuals) and spirits of camphor as a rub over the back in the region of the kidneys. These are combined with lard (mutton tallow is most often recommended), which helps open the skin's pores to allow the turpentine and cam-phor to act. These ingredients are further aided by the application of heat, often in the form of an Epsom-salt pack.

Two teas are specifically recommended to help the functioning of the liver and kidneys. Watermelon seed tea, with the diuretic saltpeter as its active ingredient, acts as a stimulant to the kidneys. And rag-weed (or ambrosia) tea is recommended as a tonic for the liver and as a laxative.

The readings have some general advice about keeping the bowel's eliminations regular. Whenever possible, dietary measures to in-crease the amount of fiber—by eating raw vegetables or prunes and decreasing the intake of meat—are the first choice. If a laxative is needed, variety is the name of the game. Fruit *and* vegetable extracts are available that stimulate peristalsis of the bowel, especially of the colon. The most mentioned laxative in the readings is Fletcher's cas-toria—made with extracts from the senna plant—which "will work with the digestive forces, the kidneys and the activities in the liver proper" (no. 786–2). This is to be taken in small and frequent doses until the desired result occurs. Eno salts, a fruit extract, and Zilatone are also recommended.

There are also mineral-based laxatives; examples are Milk of

Magnesia and citrocarbonates. These are nonabsorbable salts which draw water into the intestine by osmosis, distending it and thereby stimulating contractions. The readings recommend each of these types of laxative at different times, and more importantly, suggest that individuals rotate their use to decrease the possibility of bowel irritation or dependency.

The suggestions in this chapter should help you to maintain your eliminations and provide a better environment in which your cells can live and flourish. The benefit will be a more balanced level of energy and a clearer perspective on life—for "few may show forth that even felt in the heart with the liver bad" (no. 341–31).

9

The Rivers Within:
The Arterial and
Lymphatic Circulations

The body rebuilds itself—constantly—*through . . . the*
blood *supply.*
EDGAR CAYCE reading no. 683–3

Out of his heart shall flow rivers of living water.
JOHN 7:38

WHEN THE HEART STOPS, attempts at resuscitation are a race
against time. Prolonged curtailment of blood to the brain produces
coma and, in 6 to 8 minutes, permanent damage. Blood and the energy it carries are critical to the body. As a river nourishes the soil,
blood nourishes the organs it passes through. In this journey, our
crimson stream courses 60,000 miles, the equivalent of two-and-a-
half times around the globe, passing through every organ and past
each cell.

Imagine a tiny cell in the far reaches of your big toe. The best diet
in the world and the perfect coordination of the four eliminating systems mean little to this cell if nutrients don't reach it and wastes aren't
carried away. Under normal conditions, a laceration on the foot takes

7 to 10 days to be sufficiently healed for removing the stitches used for closure. This compares with 3 to 5 days for a cut on the face. This discrepancy in healing time comes from the difference in quantity of circulation between these two areas. If the foot is that of a diabetic whose arteries are partially blocked, further hampering the flow of blood, the cut may not heal at all. Instead, infection may set in and the foot may need to be amputated.

The readings recognize that one of the best ways to promote the healing of any condition is to improve the circulation—for "the circulation . . . is the main attribute to the physical body, or that which keeps life in the whole system" (no. 4614–1). As a result, the state of the body and the state of the blood are intimately tied together. Medicine is well along the way to fulfilling the readings' prediction that "the day may yet arrive when one may take a drop of blood and diagnose the condition of any physical body" (no. 283–2).

Most of the 60,000 miles of vessels carrying this life-giving fluid are capillaries, which form intricate, miniscule networks through all the organs and tissues. Ten capillaries laid side to side have the same diameter as a strand of hair; often red blood cells need to pass through them in single file.

Many of the capillaries remain closed much of the time. Flow through them is controlled by a structure, known as the precapillary sphincter, which operates like a sluice gate on a dam (see Figure 9-1). This structure, combined with the widening and narrowing of arteries and veins, regulates the velocity and course of the human river, instantly channeling it to where it is most needed.

This sphincter responds to changes in the blood, the nerves, and the environment. Temperature changes, emotions, mechanical stimuli such as the percussion and stroking of massage, and certain medicinal compounds are all able to affect it. As a result, it can be influenced to benefit the body.

A second parallel circulatory network is the lymphatic system. These thin, transparent vessels are even more delicate than capillaries and almost impossible to see. As a result, traditional medicine has paid little attention to them. The Cayce readings, on the other hand, indicate that this system is as important as the arterial circulation,

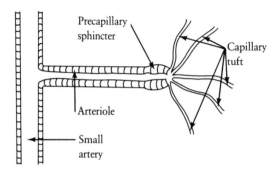

Figure 9-1.   Drawing of a precapillary sphincter.

and the readings make some fascinating observations about the role it plays in mind/body interactions (see Figure 9-2).

One role of the lymph circulation is as the garbage system of the body. The serum which flows from capillaries to bathe the cells travels a one-way street, its return prevented by a pressure gradient. As this fluid passes by them, the cells are in constant interaction with it. Nutrients are absorbed and used, waste products are expelled. Toxins, dead cells, and the by-products of cell functioning must be carried away by the lymph so that the living cells do not lose their efficiency or perish sitting in their own waste.

The challenge is to get this lymph to the liver, kidneys, lungs, and skin for processing and elimination from the body. Unlike the arterial system, the lymph does not have its own pump. There are, however, five ways to help move it through the system. Gentle massaging of these vessels with the hands or through the contraction of surrounding muscles during exercise, nerve signals stimulated with osteopathic adjustments, the application of heat and cold, and certain medicinal compounds can all enhance the circulation. Each of these five ways also helps open the precapillary sphincters, resulting in both a richer and cleaner environment for each cell to live in. Additionally, deep full breaths can act as a powerful pump for the lymph and are incorporated into many exercises suggested by the readings.

Let's take some time to look at three of these powerful techniques

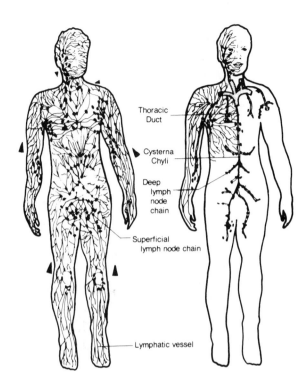

Figure 9-2. The lymphatic system.

which enhance both arterial and lymphatic flow (see Chapter 6 for a discussion of osteopathic adjustments).

EXERCISE

Active movement of our bodies can have wonderful effects. When a muscle is inactive, only a few of its capillaries are open. With exercise, up to fifty times as many may open up. Such movement can also increase lymph flow from 4 ounces an hour to 60 ounces an hour—a change of 1500 percent! You can imagine the positive effects this has on cells. It is no surprise that there is extensive research extolling the virtues of exercise.

Regular exercise causes both structural and metabolic changes in the body. The heart becomes stronger and pumps more blood with less effort, lung capacity increases, and muscles become more efficient in their use of energy. Additionally, exercise helps us stay leaner, improves sleep patterns, helps constipation, retards mineral loss from bones, and greatly improves our outlook on life. With all the evidence, it is not difficult to concur with the readings: "Exercise is wonderful, and necessary—and little or few take as much as is needed, in a systematic manner" (no. 283–1).

The readings give some specific guidelines to maximize the benefits of exercise, but in general they agree in spirit with Dr. Harold Reilly's admonition that the best exercises are "the ones that you do!" Different readings encourage tennis, golf, swimming, handball, and horseback riding. Whatever choice is made, the body needs to be prepared first by making sure it is readied for increased eliminations and by attending to known spinal lesions.

Exercise is to be started gradually and with the idea of keeping the body balanced. "To overexercise any portion not in direct need of same, to the detriment of another, is to hinder rather than to assist . . . Use common sense. Use discretion" (no. 283–1). Once started, an exercise should be continued consistently and persistently. The readings indicated a daily 5-minute walk is far better for the body than a more strenuous activity once a week. Exercise should also be approached with the correct attitude and expectancy, never as "something merely to be gotten through or gotten rid of" (no. 654–7).

An exercise program mentioned frequently in the readings includes daily walking, morning and evening setting-up exercises, head-and-neck exercises, and an abdominal exercise. Let's examine each of these.

More than once the readings indicate that walking is the best exercise of all. Walking provides the benefits mentioned above without placing too great a strain on the body. The constant movement of the legs transforms the calves into pumps that help return blood and lymph to the heart. The readings suggest that the arms be swung also to assist the upper body's circulation.

A regular time should be chosen for walking and followed rain or shine. Recommended most commonly is a walk a half hour or so after dinner. This can help rebalance the circulation, aid digestion by producing a gentle massage action on the intestines, and help relax muscles which have tightened with a day's activities—all helping to produce a more restful sleep.

To begin a walking program, set an eventual goal but start by choosing a distance you can reach comfortably. Every fourth day, increase this initial distance by 10 percent until you reach the goal you have set.

Setting-up exercises, designed to balance and equalize the circulation of the body, are recommended on arising in the morning and before bedtime. In the morning, general exercises for the upper portion of the body should be done. In the evening, general exercises from the waist down, while lying in a horizontal position, are recommended. This sequence is intended to work with naturally occurring cycles in the circulation. "The natural tendency then of the system is upper circulation, or plain activity during the day, and of body building through trunk circulation during evening" (no. 4520–4). As they help balance the circulation, setting-up exercises also help posture, the maintenance of proper weight, and the functioning of the organs.

A typical morning exercise involves slowly rising up on the toes while taking both a deep inhalation through the nostrils and gradually raising the hands above and a bit forward of the head. Then, as the body returns to standing flat on the ground, bend at the waist and swing the arms through the legs. As the hands come near the floor, forcefully expel the air from the lungs through the mouth. This is illustrated in Figure 9-3.

These movements—tightening the calf muscles, taking a deep breath using the diaphragm, and shifting the rib cage by raising the arms—help move the body's lymph. This is especially needed after its circulation has slowed during a sedentary night's rest.

The readings often advised incorporating head-and-neck exercises into the morning routine. These involve bending the head for-

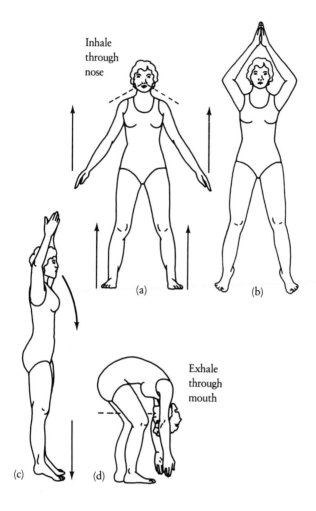

Inhale
through
nose

Exhale
through
mouth

(a)

(b)

(c)   (d)

Figure 9-3.   Typical morning exercise

ward three times, back three times, to the right three times, and to
the left three times. Then, the head is circled 360 degrees in each
direction three times. This should be done slowly, gently, and with
purpose. These head-and-neck movements are among the most recommended exercises in the readings, advocated more than three hun-

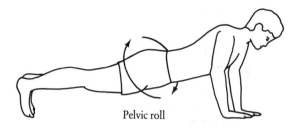

Pelvic roll

Figure 9-4.   The pelvic roll.

dred times. Their purpose is to help circulation in the head and neck area—improving vision and hearing, releasing muscular tension, and helping to relax the individual. These exercises have been valuable to many people as a prelude to meditation, although they were not directly recommended in the readings for that purpose.

For use along with the evening exercises, an abdominal exercise known as a pelvic roll is recommended. This is an exercise that "will strengthen the whole condition of the spine, keep the abdominal muscles well as to general position of the body and keep the limbs in shape . . . without being detrimental to any portion of the body" (no. 308–13). It is also supposed to help the circulation, aid digestion, and strengthen a sagging abdomen. To do this exercise, place the feet against a wall and the hands on the floor—as if preparing to do a pushup. Keeping the elbows relatively straight, circle the trunk and hips, as illustrated in Figure 9-4.

The readings warn that this exercise initially may not be easy and should be started gradually. Recommended frequency is from once a week to daily, depending on the individual.

MASSAGE

Massage is an effective technique which is often undervalued because of its simplicity. In an era obsessed with complex machinery and new techniques, the known therapeutic effects of massage deserve to be rediscovered. From the Cayce readings' perspective, the greatest values of massage are its benefits to the circulatory and nervous systems, both directly and reflexively.

Initially during massage there is contraction of the capillaries in response to the stroking pressure, followed by capillary and arteriole dilation. As a result, first blanching and then redness of the skin is observed. There is research evidence that these vascular changes affect the body. Urine production often increases for several hours after a massage; its specific gravity remains constant, indicating that solids—including uric acid, nitrogen, and phosphorus—have been mobilized and are being excreted. There is also a reported 10 to 15 percent increase in oxygen consumption and carbon dioxide production during a massage. Lymph flow is enhanced and muscle spasms are relaxed.

Massage of the back and spine has been shown to also influence the activity of the sympathetic nervous system as measured by blood pressure, pulse, temperature, pupil diameter, and respirations. Cayce reading no. 2456–4 indicates this can rebalance the nervous system as "inactivity causes many of those portions along the spine . . . to be lax, or taut . . . The massage aids the ganglia to receive impulse from nerve forces," which helps restore equilibrium.

Because of these physiological effects, the readings recommend massage for everyone. As a more specific application, a full massage should follow any technique designed to stimulate cellular eliminations (such as the use of the violet-ray applicator or Epsom-salt packs) to help move toxins to locations where they can be eliminated. A massage is also helpful after any intervention with the nervous system, such as the use of the wet-cell battery—to "wake up" the sympathetic nervous system and help it respond.

In general, there are three essential massage techniques: stroking, compression, and percussion. Stroking is a gliding motion that has a relaxing effect. Compression involves kneading and friction. Percussion incorporates cupping, slapping, and shaking. All three enhance circulation in the treated area. The same effect can be produced with an electric vibrator, often recommended for use over the spine.

The readings usually recommend the use of a massage oil. Peanut and olive oil are the most frequently cited. Peanut oil serves as a nutrient to the nerves and ganglia, the skin, and the muscles and makes each more pliable. With absorption, it also can improve the balance between the liver and the kidneys. With this ability in mind, the readings told several individuals that "those who would take a peanut oil rub each week need never fear arthritis" (no. 1158–31).

Olive oil is recommended as "one of the most effective agents for stimulating muscular activity or mucous-membrane activity, that may be applied to the body" (no. 440–3). It is regularly recommended, occasionally mixed with tincture of myrrh, for use over the spine to stimulate the superficial circulation and strengthen the muscles. For children, cocoa butter is often suggested as a substitute for olive oil and myrrh for spinal massages.

Other recommended agents include rose water, lanolin, pine needle oil, oil of sassafras, witch hazel, castor oil, camphorated oil, Russian White Oil, tincture of benzoin, and nujol. These are usually used in combination with either peanut oil or olive oil.

The formula used for general tonic massages by Dr. Reilly is:

Peanut oil	6 ounces
Olive oil	2 ounces
Lanolin, dissolved	1 tablespoon
Rose water	2 ounces

This is to be shaken well before each use.

To provide maximum benefit, a massage should be given by a trained individual and should last about an hour. However, even a short and simple self-massage can be of great value. A self-massage can stimulate the circulation, help mobilize the joints, increase flexibility, and help condition the back, shoulders, and arms at the same time.

To try this, you will need a massage oil and an ordinary bath towel. Place the towel on a carpeted floor and lie down. Throughout the massage start by lightly applying the massage oil to the area about to receive attention. Begin by choosing one limb and grasp that hand or foot, pressing your thumb(s) into the sole or palm. Massage between the bones, between the digits, and over the pads. Then, using a gentle motion, rotate each finger or toe.

Now turn your attention to the limb itself. Begin distally and work up the limb with a stroking motion. The movements, all directed toward the heart, should initially be light. With each succeeding stroke, increase the pressure. Then, with closed fist(s) gently pound the soft tissue. Return to stroking and diminish the pressure until the last stroke is light and soothing. Finish by encircling the limb with your hand(s) and milking toward the trunk in a firm and fluid movement. Move on to the next extremity, doing each one in turn.

After completing the limbs, turn your attention to the abdomen. Using a gentle rotary movement with your hand, begin in the right lower quadrant. Using these circular movements, inch your way up the right side of the abdomen to the rib cage, then across the abdomen and down the left side to the groin, following the path of the colon. Next, massage the muscles of the chest, doing one side at a time. Take care to get between each rib.

Turn your attention now to the head and scalp. First, use both hands to massage the scalp without the use of oil. Then, using your fingers in a circular motion, gently massage the sides of your nose and work outward on the cheeks to the ears. Continuing with this motion, work around the bottom of the ears and behind them. Next, rotate your head to the right and apply gentle pressure with a hand to increase your range of motion. Repeat this to the left.

Now place your hands behind your head and flex your head as far as possible toward your chest. Lay your head down again, but keep your hands behind your head and find the bump—the inion—located in the center of your lower skull. Find the vertebral spinous process directly below this and then move one inch further down your neck. You are now over the spinous process of the third vertebrae. Using your fingertips, apply deep stationary pressure here for 1 to 2 minutes. When done, work down from here on either side of the neck, once again using the same circular motion.

Now, turning on your side, twist your upper shoulder back as far as possible while bringing your upper hip and knee forward and stretch your back. Switch sides and repeat with the opposite shoulder and hip.

Finish the massage by standing and grasping the ends of the towel in each hand; work it back and forth across your back with a diagonal motion—one hand held high and the other low. Switch hand placement and repeat in the opposite diagonal. This massage will improve your circulation, increase your flexibility, and help condition you.

USE OF HEAT AND COLD

Temperature changes affect the body in a number of ways. Heat and cold influence the circulation of blood. Where heat, unless intense, is applied, blood vessels dilate. The effect of cold occurs in two steps. First, there is the primary action which, in the case of blood vessels, involves constriction. Later, there is a reaction to cold which opens the vessels and increases blood flow.

These effects on the circulation are produced in several ways. First, heat and cold both directly affect the local precapillary sphincters. While the capillaries are very small, their combined cross-sectional area is roughly eight hundred times that of the large aorta. Because of this, affecting even a portion of the capillaries can profoundly influence the body's circulation. Second, temperature affects the action of neuronal reflex arcs. The skin has millions of nerve endings that tie it in with the sympathetic nervous system, which plays a major role in controlling the circulation.

Temperature changes also affect nerve conduction velocity and the firing rate of different sensory receptors in the body, including muscle spindles. As a result of these effects, both heat and cold influence inflammatory processes, relieve muscle spasms, and increase a person's pain threshold.

The following chart summarizes the major responses of the body to heat and cold:

Heat	Cold
Vessels: dilatation	*Vessels:* constriction followed by dilatation
Muscles: increases their volume, relieves spasm	*Muscles:* reduces their volume, relieves spasm

Heat	Cold
Heart: slows and then quickens	*Heart:* quickens and then slows
Nerves: excites, speeds conduction	*Nerves:* numbs, slows conduction
Respiration: picks up	*Respiration:* slows and deepens
Gastrointestinal tract: decreases acid production, slows peristalsis	*Gastrointestinal tract:* increases acid production, quickens peristalsis
Metabolism: temporarily alkalinizes the blood by overbreathing and decreasing carbon dioxide; urea and protein waste increase	*Metabolism:* increases carbon dioxide production, temporarily acidifying the local area; improves oxidation and decreases urea
Other: increases pain threshold, decreases joint stiffness	*Other:* increases pain threshold, prevents edema and swelling following an injury

Through the neural reflexes mentioned in the chart, every organ has a reflexive relationship with the skin immediately over it. In some cases, an organ can also be affected by heat or cold applied to more distant areas. These relationships are illustrated in Figure 9-5.

The hot foot bath is an example of how these relationships can be applied. It is frequently recommended by the readings to help resolve upper respiratory and sinus problems (see Figure 9-6). Placing the feet in hot water produces a narrowing of the vessels in the head and face. As a result, the congestion of blood in the inflamed portions improves and helps increase blood flow to and away from the area.

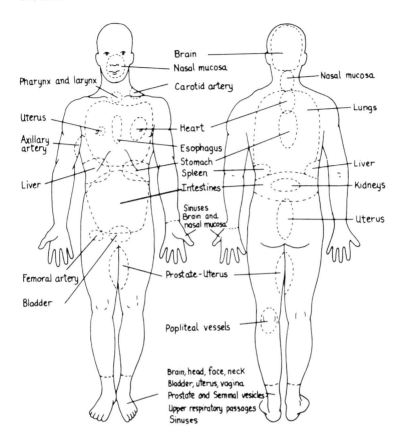

Brain
Nasal mucosa
Pharynx and larynx
Carotid artery
Nasal mucosa
Lungs
Uterus
Axillary artery
Heart
Esophagus
Stomach
Spleen
Liver
Liver
Intestines
Kidneys
Sinuses
Brain and nasal mucosa
Uterus
Femoral artery
Prostate - Uterus
Bladder
Popliteal vessels
Brain, head, face, neck
Bladder, uterus, vagina
Prostate and Seminal vesicles
Upper respiratory passages
Sinuses

Figure 9-5. Reflex areas: Apply heat or cold to the hatched areas.

Directions for a foot bath are quite simple. Use a large basin or tub and fill it with 110° F water. The readings suggest that the therapeutic effectiveness of this bath can be increased by adding 1 or 2 tablespoons of mustard to the water. The bath should last between 5 and 20 minutes. As the water cools, add more hot water.

Each of these techniques—exercise, massage, and the use of heat and cold—can help improve the body's circulation. As nutrients are carried to and wastes away from each cell, they will respond by moving toward health.

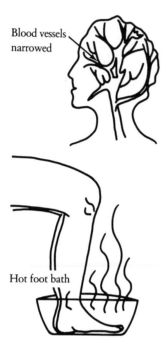

Figure 9-6.   Effects of a hot foot bath on circulation in the head region.

10

The Elusive Élan Vital: In Search of the Life Force

And he laid his hand on every one of them, and healed them.

LUKE 4:40

Know that Life itself—to be sure—is the Creative Force or God, yet its manifestations in man are electrical— or vibratory.

EDGAR CAYCE reading no. 1299–1

ALL OF US HAVE experienced lucky days when everything seems to be going our way. The Cayce readings say these are times when "there is a closer association with Creative Forces about the body" (no. 1179–1). The readings go on to describe such an association as an electrical phenomena, one which we can work directly with and influence. The readings indicate that each of us can employ measures to more fully unite our body, mind, and soul with the Trinity, a unison that helps heal the physical body.

Throughout the history of medicine and biology, individuals have searched for evidence of a physical link with the divine. This usually has involved a search for a "life force," that vital spark that would set living matter apart as being something special, more than a mere chemical phenomenon. The Hindus believed in such a force and called it *prana*; the Chinese called it *ch'i* and built their entire medical philosophy around its existence.

In the West, a litany of distinguished names—Paracelsus, van Helmont, Galvani, Volta, and Mesmer—have believed in and been in the forefront of advancing theories about such a life force. More recently, and increasingly out of the mainstream of science, other individuals—von Reichenbach, Lakhovsky, Eeman, and Reich—have spent their lives and often sacrificed their reputations in the quest. Despite such effort, the search has yielded no concrete proof.

A compelling argument against such a force was the decipherment of DNA in the 1950s. To many, this has become the ultimate proof that we have evolved during 4 billion years of chance. As science has moved forward, fewer and fewer legitimate scientists will even consider the existence of such a life force.

Their answer, however, is clearly incomplete. While biologists have shown beyond a doubt that there is a biochemistry of life, they have been unable to explain many of its most basic phenomena. The way in which our body organizes itself—such as cells aligning to form muscle, taking specific shape and having a specific relationship to bone—remains a mystery. The processes of healing, pain, sleep, and consciousness are beyond the explanation of current knowledge, as well. Biologists divide living things into smaller components for study, but, in the process, life itself slips through their fingers and all that remains is a bag of molecules. Such missing information suggests that DNA isn't the whole secret of life, but a computer program of sorts controlled by something else. Referring to this possibility, the Nobel laureate Albert Szent-Gyorgyi said, "It looks as if some basic fact about life were still missing, without which any real understanding is impossible." He suggested that biologists consider reexamining electricity as the missing piece of the puzzle.

The Cayce readings make clear that Szent-Gyorgyi's advice is excellent. According to the readings, electricity is *the* basic block upon which everything is built. "For materiality *is*—or matter *is*—that

demonstration and manifestation of the units of positive and negative energy, or electricity, or God" (no. 412–9). In other words, it is
these "units of positive and negative forces that brings it [a physical
body] into a *material* plane" (no. 281–3).

As science more closely examines the body, it encounters some
form of electricity at every turn. In the last 25 years, nearly every type
of tissue has been proven to produce or carry some kind of electrical
charge. Cells have membranes which act as insulators and allow the
creation of charge differentials between the inside of a cell and its
surrounding environment. The movement of ions across these membranes generate electrical and magnetic fields. The heart, brain, and
skeletal muscles depend on this ability to function. Medicine measures and uses these potential changes diagnostically in the form of
EKGs, EEGs, and EMGs, respectively.

Bone-forming cells are regulated by an electrical phenomenon as
well. Inorganic crystals found in the bone matrix can create an electrical field and be affected by one. As we shift our weight, these crystals change shape, producing charge differentials that stimulate bone
formation and determine the patterns in which the bone is laid down.
When immobility occurs for any reason, the bones thin, lose their
density, and are at greater risk for fracture.

At a more basic level, cell division is controlled by the electrical
voltage across the cell membrane, with increasingly negative voltages
inhibiting reproduction. In contrast to normal cells, cancer cells have
an abnormally low voltage across their membranes and, thus, prolif-
erate rapidly. Additionally, normal cells communicate electrically
through places in their membranes where the electrical resistance between them is lowered a thousand times. These areas are absent in
cancer cells, which may contribute to the lack of response they show
to the body's usual control systems.

At the prestigious Karolinska Institute in Sweden, Dr. Bjorn Nor-
denstrom has had preliminary success in treating certain cancers by
placing electrodes directly into the tumor and passing a very small
current through them.

He hypothesizes that this procedure works for several reasons.
First, he uses the positive electrode in the tumor which attracts

the primary tumor fighters of the body, electrically negative white blood cells.

Second, the charge creates an acidic environment that hampers oxygen delivery to the tumor and also affects the cancer directly.

Finally, the positive charge displaces water from the tumor, dehydrating it and causing the surrounding tissues to swell, both actions affecting the delivery of blood to nourish the cancer. (A list of the actions that the positive and negative terminals of a direct current have on living tissue is found later in this chapter.)

These are fascinating conjectures, particularly in the light of the Cayce readings' discussion of the importance of both dehydrating a tumor, creating an acidic environment at the tumor site, and the need to involve the body's immune system, when explaining the rationale of their cancer therapies.

Cells' electrical properties come into play with other common clinical occurrences as well. Sudden cardiac death can occur when part of the heart is well nourished and an adjacent part is not, forming an "oxygen differential" line. This causes a difference in the electrical potentials of the two parts, which can send the heart into fibrillation—usually a fatal occurrence.

Wound-healing is another basic example. Since the mid-nineteenth century, it has been recognized that the cell processes involved in wound-healing are accompanied by and probably depend on the formation of a current of injury, a measurable leakage of current from the wound site. Tissue repair and regeneration can be enhanced by augmenting this current with the use of external electrical stimulation. Such stimulation has also been shown to assist the healing of human fractures and ulcers, and even to partially regenerate mammalian limbs. Animals which have the ability to completely regenerate an amputated portion appear to naturally create such persistent electrical currents.

One experiment using planarian, or flatworms, which can regrow both head and tail from just a midportion, found that passing a direct current through the animal could determine at which end or ends the head would grow (see Figure 10-1).

Using such an experiment as a starting point, orthopedic surgeon

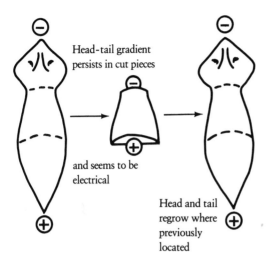

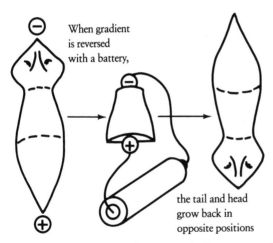

Figure 10-1. The effect of current polarity on regrowth of the planarian.

Robert Becker has made an extensive study of the process of regeneration. From this, he has postulated the existence of a direct-current electrical system in the body that flows through the perineural cells. Peri means around, and these cells, of which there are several types, form the sheaths that surround most nerves as they course through the body and also congregate around the neurons of the brain, with the result being that they actually comprise 90 percent of the brain. These cells are known to be vital for the health of neurons, which will not grow in culture unless accompanied by them.

Dr. Becker's research suggests that dc current flows through these perineural cells, separate and distinct from the neuron's better known electrochemical impulses. According to him, each neuron is electrically polarized and has a positive and a negative terminal. The cell body of the neuron, located at one end of the cell, is positively charged relative to the other end, and there is a gradual charge gradation along the neuron's length. This voltage difference becomes more negative during physical activity, declines when we sleep, and even reverses when general anesthesia is used.

Dr. Becker hypothesizes that this system may be involved in such diverse phenomena as acupuncture, hypnosis, and the mystery of pain. It may also be how the body interacts with the electromagnetic fields of the earth and sun and may help account for the body's daily and seasonal rhythms. If this is the case, the perineural system may have a special relationship with the pineal gland, which plays a role in the body's cycles. Finally, the electrical body may be involved in healing by the laying-on of hands.

Exploration of this area is still fairly new and filled with possibilities and controversy. The involved energies are real, but they are also subtle. Many of the therapies in the Cayce readings work with these energies. The premise in the readings is simple: "Electricity is life" (no. 3990–1). From the readings' perspective, the body can be viewed as a battery. The organs that maintain this battery are the heart, the lungs, the liver, and the kidneys. The latter two are often mentioned by the readings as forming the positive and negative poles of the battery.

Many of the principles already discussed in this book relate directly to maintaining the proper balance of this battery. "Toxic forces," due to improper eliminations, were said to "run down the battery for the body" (no. 3255–1). The concept of an acid-alkaline balance also has to do directly with charge and the availability of electrons in the system. Even the head-and-neck exercises and the intake of water are occasionally explained as steps to help recharge the battery forces of the body.

The role of the heart, lungs, liver, and kidneys is to maintain the proper ratios of nutrients and electrolytes within the body. For "with changes in the chemical forces of the system, [the battery] may become so reduced . . . as to cause stress . . . thus gradually building a disturbance functionally. With the distress or disturbance [thus produced,] one or the other organ gradually becomes organically disordered" (no. 4007–1). An example given by the readings of this involves fried foods and grease. The readings state that these cause a "short-circuiting" of the circulation between the heart and liver, resulting in atherosclerosis and coronary heart disease.

To directly help this battery, the Cayce readings provide directions for building a device they named the radioactive appliance. It has nothing to do with radioactivity, a term which came into usage later, so some people prefer to refer to it as the impedance device (see Figure 10-2). It consists of two pieces of carbon steel separated by glass, surrounded by carbon, and then charcoal, and finally sealed in a copper can.

To use this device, it is placed in ice water for 30 minutes to "electronize" the carbon steel. Then, its lead wires are attached to opposite limbs—the right wrist and left ankle, for example—for approximately an hour. These sessions are to be done in 4-day cycles, rotating connections to the limbs each day until all combinations have been used.

Worked with in this fashion, the impedance device is supposed to accomplish the same recuperative functions as sleep. Many people, in fact, find the device quickly causes them to enter a light sleep and the readings frequently suggest its use as a therapy for insomnia.

The Cayce readings indicate the device balances both the blood and nerve circulations. This "produces that equilibrium in the human body to relieve any tension as is caused in the deficiency or overproficiency of any electronic agent . . . Then the action is as this: An excess in one, by a unison of electronic agencies, may be forced to assist that one deficient" (no. 1800–4). Many conditions can initiate

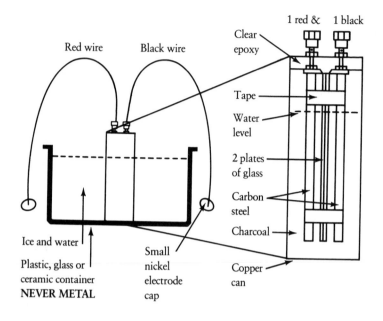

Figure 10-2. The impedance device.

such a deficiency, including injuries, infections, and lack of proper eliminations. Deficient portions of the body are unable to reproduce and rejuvenate themselves properly. The impedance device, according to the readings, assists healing by equalizing the system, but becomes curative only when assisted by the "mental forces" and the action of the "normal forces" of "appetite and rebuilding" (no. 1800–4). In the process of rebalancing the energy system, the readings say the device coordinates superficial and deeper blood circulations; improves metabolism; improves digestive forces; helps vision, taste, and hearing; and, most important, produces better coordination between the cerebrospinal and sympathetic nervous systems.

Exactly how the device works is still a mystery. Its design is that of a leaky capacitor that can collect and then evenly dispense energy. The readings say a current will never be measured passing through the leads and none has. Despite this, the readings also say that the device is not "as talismanic conditions, nor . . . the imaginations of a body, but when properly . . . constructed these correspond with the laws of physics . . . while . . . seemingly of little or no use from outward appearance" (no. 957–3).

The Cayce readings make clear that the impedance device works with "the lowest form of electrical forces" (no. 681–2). "For it is the lowest form of vibration electrically that gives creative forces, rather than the highest. It is the high vibration that destroys" (no. 933–3). (These higher vibrations are recommended for therapeutic use with the violet-ray applicator.)

The readings offer several generalizations about the device. First, its use is good for everybody, regardless of condition. Second, the device can produce states similar to meditation and the times when the impedance device is used are ideal for autosuggestion, reading spiritual material, deep thinking, visualization, and meditation. Finally, it needs to be used with expectancy, reverence, prayer, persistence, and gratitude.

While the impedance device is suggested in general conditions of circulatory or nervous system incoordination, a second appliance— the wet-cell battery—is recommended more often for specific conditons. The wet-cell battery is especially urged for ailments that involve the nervous system and glands, such as multiple sclerosis, epilepsy, Parkinson's, scleroderma, deafness, and cerebral palsy.

The wet cell is a battery consisting of metal poles in a solution of sulfuric acid, copper sulfate, zinc, willow charcoal, and distilled water (see Figure 10-3).

This setup produces a very small dc current that is weaker than that produced by a flashlight battery. Interestingly, Dr. Becker's research showed that smaller currents are often more succesful than higher levels because they approximate the natural conditions and minimize side effects.

A major component of the wet-cell battery is the solution jar. As current passes through lead loops placed in a solution, the readings indicate that the "electronic energies partake" of the solution's vibration as it "decomposes." This apparently affects the vibratory rate of the current and relays a message to the body.

The readings make fascinating references to how this informa-

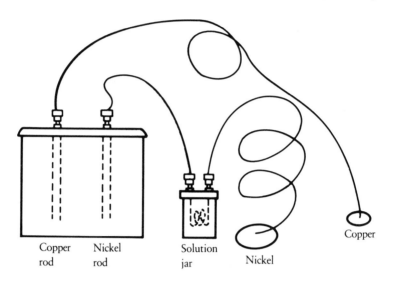

Figure 10-3. Wet-cell battery.

tion is transferred to and works within the body. Most often, the wire leads from the wet cell are attached with the negative pole—the one carrying the altered vibration—to the area just above and to the right of the umbilicus. The readings give three reasons for this location. First, any external vibration is best received in the area where the embryo received its nourishment. While the "blood centers have been closed . . . the nerve vibrations may be re-opened by same" (no. 1800–11). Second, this location is stated to be the center of the body's energy circulation, which is in the form of a figure eight. Finally, this area is also referred to as the solar plexus center, which the readings describe as the center of our nervous system.

In using the wet-cell battery, the positive pole is usually placed over the spine. The locations most frequently recommended are the areas where, according to the readings, the cerebrospinal and sympathetic nervous systems and the lymphatic system all maximally interact. These four areas are the second through fourth cervical, the second through fourth dorsal, the ninth dorsal, and the second through fourth lumbar.

Applied properly, the wet-cell battery is supposed to work by awakening the subconscious (the autonomic nervous system) to help supply the body with the element in the solution jar. To help us understand this, the readings compare it with how our body responds to watching someone else eat. The visual and olfactory input causes both the release of gastric juices and stomach contractions. These signals are relayed to our consciosness and interpreted as hunger. In a similar fashion, the vibrations entering the umbilical center bring to the attention of the subconscious the need to fulfill a certain hunger.

A number of solutions were used in this jar. The one most commonly recommended is gold chloride, said to help the glands and nervous system with "rejuvenating any organ of the system showing the delinquency in action" (no. 1800–6). Also, recommended frequently are silver nitrate, spirits of camphor, and tincture of iodine.

The dc current itself also can directly affect the body. The following table lists the actions produced at the respective poles:

Positive Pole	**Negative Pole**
Repels bases, tissue becomes acidic	Repels acids, tissue becomes alkaline
Dehydrates tissues	Swells tissue
Produces vasoconstriction, causing ischemia and stopping bleeding	Produces vasodilatation, causing hypermia and bleeding
Attracts oxygen	Attracts hydrogen
Sedative	Stimulant

The Cayce readings recommended a third device, the violet-ray applicator, a high-voltage, low-amperage source of static electricity. It should not be confused with ultraviolet light. Its name comes from the color of the electrical discharge which emanates from a glass applicator. Static electricity has a long history in healing, associated with such men as Benjamin Franklin, Marat of the French Revolution, and John Wesley.

Unlike the two devices described earlier, the violet-ray applicator was not invented by the readings; most American medical practitioners at the turn of the century had static electricity machines in their offices.

The readings describe the violet-ray as employing the "higher forces" or ones "destructive" to the body. Its role is to break down, not build up, the tissue. Most often the device was used to break up firmly entrenched conditions at a specific site so they could be eliminated from the body.

These three devices are not widely used. Many of their effects are subtle and their operating principles are often difficult to understand, based on our current knowledge. They may, however, be a vital piece in the puzzle of understanding how our bodies work. We *are* electromagnetic beings and this is perhaps the clearest physical connection we have with God. Knowledge and application in this entire area needs to be pursued further.

11

The Next Step:
Longevity and Regeneration

*It is not what one knows that counts, but what one does
about that it knows!*
EDGAR CAYCE reading no. 1182–1

*If to do were as easy as to know what were good to do,
chapels had been churches, and poor men's cottages
princes' palaces.*
WILLIAM SHAKESPEARE, The Merchant of Venice

A REPEATED THEME IN the myths and literature of many cultures
is the search for a "fountain of youth." This preoccupation with longevity was often reflected in the questions that were asked of Cayce.
Some fascinating answers were the result. A 42-year-old-man asked
how long he would live in this incarnation and was told, "To a hundred and fifty!" (no. 866–1). Others were told that they could live to
be 120 years old—if they lived right, ate properly, and kept their
mental outlook creative and optimistic. Reading no. 244–2 advised
"Man should live much longer than has been ordinarily given—and
will!"

Science agrees with the Cayce perspective. Research shows that all of life seems to have a built-in longevity clock. Fruit flies live approximately forty days, mice 3 years, and horses 30 years. Using a number of methods, many scientists have guessed that our "normal" life span should approach 120 years of age.

In Hunza, the Vilcabamba valley of Ecuador, and the Caucasus, there are models of societies where longevity is the rule, not the exception, and individuals regularly live to more than 100 years of age. Given ideal conditions in a laboratory, human fibroblast cells have lived for sixty or more cycles, the equivalent of a 150-year life span.

The Cayce readings go beyond even these predictions. Paralleling biblical stories of lifespans approaching 1,000 years, they make clear that if our days were numbered by anything—including a biological clock—it would be a violation of our free will. Our life is limited only by our choices and expectations. The promise of rejuvenation is real. "For, the ability . . . to reproduce itself . . . keeps [the body] not only young but active—mentally, spiritually, physically—unless it be drugged by its own ego" (no. 3042–1).

The promise of long life, however, comes with a stipulation: "One may preserve youth, even as is desired, will they pay the *price* as is *necessary* (no. 900–465). For "the body is the most adaptable institution that is manifested in the earth; yet it is so easily abused" (no. 1158–31).

Paying a price for health and longevity runs against our hope for a quick and easy approach. Many early searches for eternal youth looked for magical answers. Alchemists sought the instant transformation of "lead to gold" as an archetype for their own transmutation. Ponce de Leon searched high and low for a way to make immortality as easy as a drink of water.

The Cayce readings place a few such carrots before us. Turtle eggs are confirmed as helping extend the usefulness of certain cells. Gold and silver, if used properly, are stated to carry the potential of doubling our life span.

The core of the Cayce readings, however, do not suggest a magical approach. "Regeneration may not come about by merely injections of extracts or compounds to react, but must be as a gradual growth of the expression and coordination of the nervous systems and the physical reactions to creative and generative forces within the body-functionings themselves" (no. 2248–1). This path requires more than magic; it requires basic lifestyle changes.

Making changes in the way we think, act, and feel can be a tremendous challenge. Bernie Siegel, M.D., notes that if he gave the cancer patients with whom he works the choice of either changing their lifestyle or having an operation, most would say, "Operate, it hurts less."

Change requires commitment, awareness, assessment, action, and patience. Let's examine these one at a time.

The first step in this process is making the decision that health *is* a priority. How much time we spend on something directly reflects our level of commitment to it. Health habits, like any other important event, need to be scheduled into the day. Make the time for them before the time is made for you.

As we make a commitment for change, we should consider the factors motivating us to do so. A 59-year-old woman asked how many more years of life she could expect. In response, the Cayce reading make clear the relationship between purpose and its effect on life span.

> How many do you wish? Let the prayer be ever: 'Father, so long as I may be useful as a manifestation of Thy love in the earth, and as I may be gentle and kind and true and pure to my fellow man, keep Thou, O Lord, me.' (no. 4055–2)

The readings are even more direct in the question they posed to another individual: "What need is there for a better body, [except] to serve thy fellow man the better?" (no. 1620–1). Longevity should be a welcomed side effect, not our intent. Our reasons for desiring health should not be self-serving.

Commitment is required to map out an *individualized* approach to health. The readings emphasize that each person is a unique composite of mind and body. We all share the same Spirit, but we personalize its manifestations. The Cayce readings stress our individuality: "In giving a discourse upon how this entity may extend the life expectancy, . . . each soul, is in many respects a law unto itself; especially as related to the activities and the diets that would extend or impel life expectancy" (no. 2533–6). In short, any program must be tailored to our specific individual needs.

We need to develop healthful self-awareness in order to begin to understand our unique needs. Fritz Perls, the originator of Gestalt therapy, noted that "Awareness per se—by and of itself—can be curative." Attuning the physical and mental with the spiritual in our journey toward wholeness is greatly facilitated by such awareness.

There are several ways to develop a health awareness. One is to take time daily to do an activity with your full attention, be it a breathing exercise or brushing your teeth. With practice, this focused mindfulness will start spilling over into other areas of your life. As we become more aware of our body and are willing to listen to it, we can respond to its needs more appropriately.

Another way to develop more of an awareness is to keep a journal. Such a journaling experience might include dream work, health tracking, spiritual reading, and working with disciplines. The format for this can be done any number of ways; exact emphasis should grow out of one's own needs. One style that could be used is given in Figure 11-1.

A simple suggestion in the Cayce readings is to record the experiences of each day on paper at bedtime. "Not to be studied, not to be exploited or shown or given to others, but for self! And *do not* read same after it is written for at least 30 days. And then note the difference in what you are thinking . . . , what your desires are, what your experiences are!" (no. 830–3). As you work with a journal to improve your level of awareness, try the following exercise. Focus on the eight concepts listed below, one at a time, for 3 to 7 days each. Detach and observe your approach and behavior toward your body and see if these are compatible with the following statements:

1. We are spiritual beings. The body is the temple of the soul and the dwelling place of the mind.
2. There is a pattern within every system of the body for the proper functioning of the cells of that system.

3. Each part, each structure, each system of the body affects and bears a relationship to the whole.
4. *We* are responsible for the bodies we have built and are building.
5. Attitudes affect the physical body and do so constructively or destructively.
6. The system is builded by the assimilations that it takes within and is able to bring resuscitation so long as the eliminations do not hinder.
7. Rest and recreation are spiritual, mental, and physical necessities.
8. Application must be persistent and consistent.

(From the Association for Research and Enlightenment's "Thirty Days to a Healthier You" home-study course.)

From an improved awareness will emerge the opportunity for a more thorough and accurate assessment of how your body works and what its needs are. Such analysis occurs at many levels. First, it can and should occur at a very logical and analytical level:

> Do not believe in anything merely because it is said, nor in traditions because they have been handed down from antiquity; nor in rumors as such; nor in writings by sages because sages wrote them; nor in fancies we suspect to have been inspired in us by a Deva; nor in inferences drawn from some haphazard assumption we may have made; nor in what seems to be an analogical necessity; nor in the mere authority of our teachers and masters. Believe when the writing, doctrine, or saying is corroborated by reason and consciousness.
> GAUTAMA BUDDHA

The more you know of your own body's physiology and anatomy, the better you will be at this task.

Also helpful at this level is a good relationship with a medical doctor who can serve as an adviser and a source of information. Here are some ideas on what constitutes an optimal interaction with a doctor:

• First, expect less. The primary responsibility for your health belongs to you. Know your body and understand your ailment

Spiritual Verse

"I appeal to you therefore, brethren, by the mercies of God, to present your bodies as a living sacrifice, holy and acceptable to God, which is your spiritual worship. Do not be conformed to this world, but be transformed by the renewal of your mind, that you may prove what is the will of God, what is good and acceptable and perfect."

Romans 12:1–2

Daily Disciplines

	Mon.	Tues.	Wed.	Thurs.	Fri.	Sat.	Sun.
Meditate	√	√					
Noon Salad		√					
A.M. Exercise	√	√					
P.M. Exercise	√						
8 Glasses Water	√						
Spiritual Reading	√						

Weekly Goals

One day of minimal talk ☑
Memorize spiritual verse ☐
Health: Order impedance device ☐
    Schedule colonic ☑
    Work to personalize the exercises ☐

Dream Journal

Monday, 7/17— In the dream, I was standing on the porch of an old house. . . .

Daily Review

Tuesday, 7/18—Today I found myself struggling with inner feelings about what direction I should take in my job situation. . . .

Figure 11-1. Sample journal page.

as much as you can. Don't depend on your doctor for all of your information.

- Move away from the "magic bullet" concept. It is estimated that seventy-five percent of the patients who visit their family doctor have conditions that will get better on their own, if they get better at all. If you go to your doctor because you want a prescription, you'll get one (often for a drug to make you feel psychologically better, like Valium).

- Remember where your healing really comes from.

  "For who healeth all thy diseases? If ye think it is the doctor or the surgeon, who is thy doctor? Is his life different from your own?" (3684–1)

- Look for a doctor who communicates with you, even if you don't completely agree with his or her approach. One of a doctor's most valuable roles is helping you understand what might and might not help and your doctor should be willing to discuss the different options available to you. Your doctor should serve as a facilitator, not a god, in your quest for health. Most doctors, like everyone else, are good folk doing their best, but they may sometimes give you the opportunity to work on patience.

- Find a balance between realizing your doctor's humanness and empowering your relationship with them. There can and should be power in your interaction. Your attitude and beliefs can help or hinder your healing and your doctor can influence these. Once you have chosen a therapy, be it surgery or castor oil, go with it wholeheartedly and empower it.

Assessment can also occur at an intuitive level. The readings indicate that hunches are worth pursuing if we are working with our spiritual ideal. Information may come to us through our meditation and dream work or in the form of a strong feeling about something. As we increase our awareness, this intuitive aspect of our assessment ability will especially be strengthened.

The "self-reading" that follows can be helpful in eliciting information at the intuitive level. Adapted from the A.R.E.'s home-study course, "Thirty Days to a Healthier You," it is formatted is a style similar to the Cayce readings. Pick a time to complete this when you are relaxed, not hurried, and feeling in touch with your body; following a period of meditation and prayer might be ideal. Don't take time to ponder each answer—proceed fairly quickly and write the first response that occurs to you.

SELF-READING

This psychic reading given by myself in _____

(location), this _____ day of _____ , 19 __ , in accordance with request made by self.

    Yes, we have the body.

    As we find, while there are many conditions that are very good in many respects, physically and mentally, there are some hindrances the correction of which would make for a better condition in the physical and prevent disturbances later that might become very disturbing without the corrections in the present.

    What are the disturbing factors and the conditions in *this* physical body?

    First, there is the feeling at times of _____

and the inability to _____ . We find

also that at times those periods when _____ .
These are the things that disturb this body.

    But, as the conditions have been created in the body and the disturbances are a fact, what *now* is to be done about these conditions?

    As we find, these we would do in the present:

    First, as to the attitude. Keep in the mental attitude of _____

_____ . Let there not be any _____

nor _____ . Then, we would also add

to the mental diet this one thing: _____ .
We find too, that the activities should be governed by the proper association of diet; for that upon which the body feeds it becomes.

    Keep away from _____ and

———————————————————————— . Do have often ———————

————————————————————— .

Budget the time so that there may be a regular period for sustaining the physical being and also for sustaining the mental and spiritual being. You are not giving sufficient time to ————————————————————————— and ————————————————————————— in the present.

To change this and bring about better conditions, we find you should start now to ————————————————————————— . Do this consistently and persistently. Later then it would also be well if you would

————————————————————————— .

Doing these things, as we find, will bring for this body, in the present experience, a contentment. And contentment does not mean being satisfied; but know by the life the body lives, the things the body thinks it desires to do for those about the self that aid in its activity, it will bring those consciousnesses of a life worthwhile, and experience that can bring material and mental and spiritual comprehension and satisfaction.

Ready for questions:

Q-1. What exercise would be well for this body?

A-1. Well that each day the body ————————————————————————— .

Q-2. How can I overcome the nerve strain and tension I'm under at times?

A-2. For this particular body this can best be done by ———————————

————————————————————— .

Q-3. How might I improve the quality of my life at this time?

A-3. Do have periods from time to time when you ———————————

————————————————————————— just for the fun of doing so.

Q-4. What is it I sometimes do to sabotage myself to keep from accomplishing what I want to do?

A-4. This entity knows that you sometimes ———————————————

————————————————————————— and this prevents the better expression.

We are through for the present.

Once commitment, awareness, and assessment are well under way, it is time for action. If we want to learn how to play a musical instrument, we need to do more than just read how it is done. Knowledge helps, but at some point the student needs to actually pick up the instrument and make a go of it. The same principle applies to our bodies. Sooner or later we need to make the step from passive observer to active student and begin to consciously interact with the instrument we were born playing.

As you gather information with your assessment, set goals for your journey to better health. Review the "ABCs of Health" in Chapter Two. The concepts of application, balance, working the body's cycles, consistency and persistency, expectancy, and taking time to relax and play are all valuable. Include your entire being—spiritual, mental, and physical—as you map your goals and how you intend to achieve them. As the chapters in this book have emphasized, this necessitates choosing a spiritual ideal, incorporating meditation and other techniques to help transform your patterns, and working with your current emotional being. In addition, working to balance your nervous system with osteopathic manipulations is very important. At a very practical level, each cell in your body needs assistance to get the necessary building blocks and rid itself of poisons. This involves the four-step process of proper diet and nutrition, getting the nutrients to the cell via the bloodstream, speeding wastes away (mainly in the lymphatic system), and finally, disposing of these wastes through one of the four eliminating systems. As we've noted, this formula for action forms the basis of all the practical therapies suggested in the Cayce readings. As we follow these, there is the promise of renewal and regeneration starting at the level of the cell.

To help you assess how you are doing at incorporating these concepts into your life, take a few minutes now to calculate your Cayce Quotient (CQ), Figure 11.2. Use your score as a feedback system and work to improve it over time.

One question that often arises in choosing a course of action is *What is the proper use of medication and surgery?* In this age, the words *drugs, medicine,* and *healing* are often synonymous. If the body is constantly renewing itself, is there a need for medicine at all?

Figure 11-2: My Cayce quotient.

No or never	Rarely	Some-times	Often	Yes or usually	
0	1	2	3	4	
—	—	—	—	—	1. I avoid fried foods.
—	—	—	—	—	2. I get 7–8 hours of sleep a night.
—	—	—	—	—	3. I do some form of stretching or limbering for 10–20 minutes daily.
—	—	—	—	—	4. I drink 6–8 glasses of water daily.
—	—	—	—	—	5. I work with my dreams.
—	—	—	—	—	6. I chew my food well and eat slowly.
—	—	—	—	—	7. I have a colonic at least twice a year.
—	—	—	—	—	8. Three-fourths of my diet consists of fruits and vegetables.
—	—	—	—	—	9. I rarely eat red meat.
—	—	—	—	—	10. I get my spine adjusted regularly.
—	—	—	—	—	11. I use the apple diet for inner cleaning at least once a year.
—	—	—	—	—	12. I am familiar with how and when to use a castor oil pack and do so.
—	—	—	—	—	13. I meditate or do some form of specific relaxation exercise for 20 minutes daily.
—	—	—	—	—	14. I know my spiritual ideal and base my decisions about my body on it.
—	—	—	—	—	15. I eat a salad and/or other raw vegetables daily.
—	—	—	—	—	16. I have some form of mild daily exercise, like walking, which I keep up regularly.
—	—	—	—	—	17. I consciously try to make three other people laugh a day.
—	—	—	—	—	18. I know how and when to use the impedance device and do so.
—	—	—	—	—	19. I drink less than three cups of coffee or tea a day and never use cream with it.
—	—	—	—	—	20. I know the value of different massage oils and use them on myself regularly.
—	—	—	—	—	21. I have abundant expectancy and visualize my body the way I want it regularly.
—	—	—	—	—	22. I perceive problems as steppingstones and not stumbling-stones.

(continued)

Figure 11-2:   My Cayce quotient (continued).

No or never	Rarely	Some-times	Often	Yes or usually		
0	1	2	3	4		
—	—	—	—	—	23.	I am aware when I am responding to a set "internal tape" and can alter my actions accordingly.
—	—	—	—	—	24.	I use positive thoughts and attitudes to affect how things happen in my life.
—	—	—	—	—	25.	I have used presleep suggestions and/or self-hypnosis to improve my health.

_____Total Score

Scoring: 85–100—You should be writing this book.
      50–85—You already know quite a bit about Cayce or alternative health
             concepts and are working to apply what you know.
      25–55—You are either a hard-working beginner or a lazy old-timer.
Less than 25—Time to get to work.

The readings' position is that drugs, like any other physical application, can help facilitate the healing process by "giving the incentive" to an ailing body.

Most of the drugs now available have appeared in the past 30 years, long after Cayce gave his last readings. However, there were medications existing in the 1920s, 1930s, and 1940s on which the readings did comment. From these comments, we can draw some conclusions that apply to the newer drugs as well.

Drugs were *not* the preferred therapy in the readings, but the Cayce source often told individuals to continue their medications and, on occasion, spontaneously recommended their use. As with most things, the Cayce readings presented a balanced approach to this topic, and drugs were recognized as having the potential to aid the healing process.

The proper role of a medicine is to "create a different element of consciousness in the system"(no. 331–1) so as to make "it aware of its relationship to the spiritual or God-force" (no. 2812–1).

To do this, medicines mimic the body's own natural processes. Drugs act on receptors which exist naturally in the body. A classic example is morphine. Morphine communicates its message by attaching to specific receptors which exist on cell membranes. It struck researchers that those receptors had not been created in anticipation of the purification of morphine from the poppy plant in 1803. They must exist because the body has its own molecule that can attach to them. In the mid-1970s, scientists went searching within the body and discovered endorphins. This same reasoning applies to all medicines active in the body.

"If an application . . . is helpful, mis-applied it must be harmful—this is natural!" (no. 1179–3). This generalization certainly includes drugs. The Cayce readings give at least three ways in which medicine can be harmful:

- It may act directly as a poison in its method of action.
- Indirectly, its action may hamper other normal processes.
- More subtly, and at a different level, a drug can give the illusion of healing when in fact it is just blocking symptoms and acting as a palliative. And "palliatives may be injected for a time; but half a truth is worse than a whole lie, for it deceiveth even the soul!" (no. 366–1).

Two examples with common drugs help illustrate this. The readings indicate that sedatives "tie up" the activities of the glands and "dull" the responses of the body. When used for any extended period, they "must become destructive to the better functioning of the body" (no. 1264–1). Likewise, the use of aspirin for rheumatoid arthritis is recognized by the readings as helping with the pain and inflammation. In the process, however, it also deadens the nerves of the gut, hampering the body's ability to work fully with assimilation and eliminations, and carries the potential of slowing real healing.

The following are some general guidelines which can be used to make decisions regarding the use of a medication:

- "The less medications . . . the better it will be for the body; provided these are not necessary to add stimulation . . . or for the strengthening of the body" (no. 1173–5).
- Look beyond the immediate goal of symptom relief. In one

reading Cayce gave for himself, a question was asked about how his condition could be relieved at once. The response was that narcotics could be used to deaden the nerve action. This was not the best option though, that it would be better to treat that which was producing the pain. In other words, pain relief did not correspond with getting to the root of the problem.

- The optimal use of a drug is for short-term assistance while the body is being rebalanced with nutrition, improved eliminations, and coordination of the nervous and glandular systems.

- Follow the principles of cycling and always taper off from medicine slowly—don't shock the body with any sudden withdrawal. The ideal role of medicine is to reawaken in the body the memory of how to produce the same influence itself. The idea is that "nature's storehouse (thine own body) may be induced to create every influence necessary for bringing greater and better and nearer normal conditions" (no. 1309–1).

- When the decision is made to take a medicine, think positive: for "their [drugs] activity are aided the more by the *correct* or proper *attitude*" (no. 464–13). To quote Bernie Siegel, M.D., "The most important thing for people to do is enter the therapy of their choice with a positive attitude."

- As you take drugs, visualize them working in harmony with the body and having the desired effect. "See them as they are being taken, or as they are being administered, creating an attunement with the Divine within" (no. 1151–5).

Similar questions can be asked regarding surgery. If each cell is so critical to the body and its functioning, what should the role of surgery be?

The readings saw surgery as a last resort, apparently keeping a number of people off the operating table with their suggestions. The premise was that operations are not necessary unless the condition has been allowed to reach the point where the cells have created a new activity separate from the rest of the body.

When this activity occurred, however, the readings did not hesitate to recommend surgery. For comparison, they use the analogy of a rotten apple, which if "left in a barrel may make all of these rotten

[and] no matter how many sound ones are put about it, the rotten one will never be made sound" (no. 243–7). As an example, individuals with an operable cancer were often told to go see a surgeon immediately.

As we travel this journey to wholeness, the final ingredient is patience. The Cayce readings tell us that through patience we will gain our souls. Our bodies present a perfect opportunity to learn patience. Consistent and persistent application is often required for any permanent change or cure at the spiritual, mental, or physical levels.

We need to remember that health is a process. We may not always experience immediate results as we apply what we know to do. But if we chart a course toward health and pursue it in earnest, our final destination is not critical. Even if a chronic illness persists, or a cancer finally overwhelms our defenses, we will have begun the ultimate journey toward wholeness.

PART II

Applying the Cayce Paradigm

12

Summaries of Cayce's Treatments

THE FIRST PART OF this book presents the general concepts and basic therapies of the Cayce physical readings. This section presents the readings' approach to fifteen varied conditions, ranging from coronary artery disease, which will affect the vast majority of us, to epilepsy and schizophrenia.

In each case, the outlines summarize the readings' perspective on the causes and treatment of the condition. *All* the readings on a given topic were reviewed and a compilation of their information put together. As you'll see, the readings approach each condition with the perspective of both balancing the body with general measures as well as applications directed at the specific factors causing the problem. The treatments are not random or magical, but are consistent, orderly, and directed at the etiology proposed by the readings. While the treatment section focuses on physical measures that were recommended, it should be clearly understood that the spiritual and mental principles discussed in Part One apply to each and every one of these fifteen conditions.

Unlike Part One, these outlines are not intended for general consumption. Their language is technical and they are not always self-explanatory. Occasionally, they assume a knowlege of the anatomy or physiology of the condition and/or a willingness to spend the time researching the condition further—perhaps because of a vested interest in understanding it better.

Many of these therapeutic regimens have not been used clinically on a regular basis and none has been adequately researched. Many of the concepts make sense with what we know; others are quite novel. Any attempt to follow these should be done under the care and advice of a health practitioner. While it is important to work with your body, that is not synonymous with playing games with it. Hopefully, over time, more experience will be gained with these regimens and they will be further refined and improved.

ALCOHOLISM

Overview

1. Defined as any drinking which causes recurring trouble—whether interpersonal, medical, financial, legal, or occupational. It is associated with a wide array of medical illnesses, leaving no organ system unaffected and more than doubling the death rate of affected persons (compared with the nonalcoholic population of the same age).

2. Alcoholism ranks among the top three causes of death and disability in the U.S., along with cardiovascular diseases and cancer.

3. It is one of the most treatable of all medical and psychiatric conditions with about a 70 percent long-term success rate, but three-fourths of all alcoholics do not receive treatment.

Causes

1. The cause of alcoholism appears to involve many factors—physical, psychological, and social—which interact in ways which are poorly understood.

2. The Cayce readings agree that there is no single cause and that each case had its own blend of problems.

3. In many, the addiction represents a strong desire pattern or habit embedded in the sympathetic nervous system (see Chapter Three) which "possesses" the individual.

4. This physical memory appears to be present or "inherited" in at least half of all alcoholics prior to drinking in this lifetime and is a strong predisposing factor.

Treatment

1. The major goal of treatment is to achieve and maintain abstinence, as the desire pattern is easily reactivated.

2. The most effective treatment options commonly available are the Alcoholics Anonymous program (which combines a spiritual growth approach with the strong social support of other ex-alcoholics), counseling or psychotherapy, and Antabuse (a drug which acts as a deterrent to drinking by making the individual feel very ill when they consume alcohol).

3. The Cayce readings emphasize this approach as well:

   a. Long-term success depends on a change in the psyche and attitude; to accomplish this, a spiritual approach involving prayer and Bible reading are recommended.

   b. Formal counseling and a stay at a treatment center are recommended for some individuals.

   c. In more than half the cases in the readings, one of two medicinal approaches is suggested: either the use of gold in oral form combined with bromide of soda or with the use of the wet-cell battery (it is stated the gold will help change the desire pattern in the nervous system), or the use of a "chemical fence" to discourage drinking (like Antabuse) consisting of oil of eucalyptus, oil of turp, and compound of tincture of benzoin.

4. General osteopathic treatments to help coordinate the nervous system.

5. Work with general dietary improvement

ASTHMA

Overview

1. Characterized by recurrent attacks of coughing, shortness of breath, and wheezing caused by spasm of the bronchial smooth muscle, swelling of the surrounding cells, and accumulation of thick mucus.
2. Affects 5 percent of the population at some point in their lives, either as children or as adults.
3. Attacks can be precipitated by a large number of diverse stimuli including allergens, cold air, emotional stress, pollutants, and certain drugs.
4. Traditional medicine divides asthma into intrinsic and extrinsic (or allergic) varieties; however, 80 percent of asthmatics have a component of both and so the division is somewhat artificial.

Causes

1. Traditional medicine has yet to propose a unifying theory on how all the varied stimuli can produce an attack; both neural reflex's and immune cells in the lung tissue are believed to play a role.
2. The Cayce readings suggest that a single mechanism underlies the vast majority of asthmatic attacks—namely, "spinal lesions" and a facilitated neural reflex (see Chapter Six), most commonly in the upper dorsal region; factors producing these lesions include injuries, sometimes occurring at birth, and previous lung infections.
3. With the balance between the central and sympathetic nervous systems disrupted, any number of factors can further place pressure on the system and trigger the neural reflex causing bronchial

constriction; the readings make some interesting observations about how these act:

a. Cold, heat, sweets, pollen, and dust are agents cited as being able to directly irritate the sympathetic nervous system through the mucous membranes of the throat, nasal passages, larynx, bronchi, and lungs (valid in light of research showing pollen is too large to reach the airways where they are supposed to act).

b. The readings implicate this same neural reflex even in clear cases of allergic asthma (and again, research shows that when an antigen-antibody complex was introduced into one lung, bronchospasm occurred in both lungs).

c. Poor eliminations, upper respiratory infections, and diet can all produce an "over-acidity" of the system which can hypersensitize the system and provoke an attack.

d. Worry and anxiety are specifically mentioned as emotions which could worsen the condition.

e. Barometric changes in the atmosphere are stated to affect the ganglia of the nervous system; the worst combination for asthmatics is a combination of humidity with a low barometric pressure.

f. Some individuals were said to have such sensitive sympathetic nervous systems that odors or even suggestions could disrupt the balance

Treatment

1. Osteopathic adjustments are recommended as the single therapy which can produce long-term improvement; most commonly with an emphasis on the upper dorsal region, often working to coordinate better with either the cervical or the lumbar vetebrae.

2. The following are recommended for use with an acute attack:

   a. Calcidin (no longer available) and/or Atomidine

   b. An inhalant used with a wide mouth jar; the formulas varied but a typical one was to use 4 ounces of pure grain alcohol as the base and add the following in the order named—oil of eucalyptus (20 drops), rectified oil of turpentine (5 drops), and compound tincture of benzoin (15 drops).

3. Follow the diet recommended in Chapter Seven with an emphasis on avoiding refined sweets and eating more vegetables that grow above the ground.

4. Improve elimination patterns, especially with the use of occasional colonics or enemas.

5. Occasionally, a move to a sunnier climate and/or a higher altitude was recommended as a temporary measure while the osteopathic adjustments were being obtained.

CANCER

Overview

1. Represents a common group of diseases—about 800,000 new cases are diagnosed in the U.S. each year; the readings state that there are nineteen variations of cancer.

2. All cancers are characterized by the uncontrollable growth of cells originating from normal tissues which eventually kill the host by local or distant spreading; the readings describe cancer as cells which establish "an organism in itself"; the cancer exists "of its *own* resuscitation, living upon the life of the body-physical."

3. Cancer cells often resemble nondifferentiated fetal cells which communicate less with and adhere less to other cells; they do not respond to normal control mechanisms and have been shown to be capable of living indefinitely in a laboratory culture dish.

Causes

1. Traditional medicine holds that cancer originates from a combination of genetic, dietary, environmental factors (such as chemicals and radiation), and exposure to certain viruses.

2. The Cayce readings agree that cancerous conditions can occur at sites where there is some form of irritation combined with hindered or unbalanced elimination patterns—and cancer, in fact, does occur more often where there is need for more cell repair at sites of constant irritation or metaplasia; certain areas of our body are more disposed to this than others based on inherited predispositions.

3. The malignancy is stated by the readings to actually arise from "broken cellular tissue."

4. For the cancer to initially develop, "the leucocyte" or immune system needed to be functioning suboptimally—mental worry, overtaxation physically, diet, impaired eliminations, and a superacidity of the tissues could all contribute to this.

Treatment

1. The approach to the treatment of cancer by the Cayce readings is unique for the readings—these cells were viewed as a separate organism and something to be warred against and gotten rid of, instead of the usual attempt to coax the cells back into working with the whole.

2. Thus there are two options—(a) if the cancer is contained and operable then surgery is often recommended, or (b) a consistent and persistent attempt to absorb the cancer is suggested by strengthening the immune system so that it can eliminate the cancer cells.

3. Either way, it is recommended to first prepare the system to eliminate properly before "scattering" the tumor; to accomplish this, osteopathic manipulations and proper diet are recommended.

4. To help vitalize the functioning of the immune system's tumor surveillance system, specific dietary suggestions are made: the elimination of all red meats and fried foods, the consuming of less oils and fats, and making the diet more alkaline than usual with lots of raw vegetables; beef juice, cod-liver oil, and liver extract, as well as foods with lots of vitamin B-1—especially

fruits and vegetables which are yellow in color—are specifically mentioned as helping stimulate the leucocytes; almonds are said to contain a "form of vitamin" that would help prevent cancer if eaten daily.

5. A number of innovative therapies are suggested by the readings; by far the most commonly mentioned is the use of carbon ash taken internally by placing it on the tongue and washing it down with water; 30 to 40 minutes later, specific areas of the body are exposed to ultraviolet light (sometimes over the area of the cancer, but just as often over the corresponding area of the spine), which apparently creates a photosensitive activation of the carbon ash causing an increase in tissue oxygenation with a corresponding activation of leucocytes and dehydration of tumor tissue; a green glass is sometimes placed between the ultraviolet light and the body to soften the effect of the ultraviolet light and to transmit a healing green color to the cells; occasionally, for superficial cancers, the ash is combined with iodine in an ointment base and applied locally.

6. Plantain tea is recommended as an adjunct for internal cancers; it is also suggested as a salve in which the leaves are cooked together with sweet cream and then applied to the areas surrounding (but not on) skin lesions or palpable lymph nodes; this is said to help dry the cancer and keep it localized.

7. Other treatments that are occasionally recommended, all with the apparent intention of stimulating the immune system to function better, are the use of "wolve" or niccolite, atropine used with the impedance device, and several methods for culturing an individual's blood to activate the immune cells or injecting an animal with the cancer cells and using their serum for local application.

8. Occasionally, the use of the magnetic effect of the laying on of hands or the actual use of a large magnet is recommended.

9. For pain, instead of using narcotics, the following ingredients placed in a capsule and taken once a day are recommended: oil of eucalyptol (1 minim), codeine (1/80 grain), rectified oil of turp

(1/2 minim), and oil of pine (1/2 minim). While this contains a small amount of a narcotic, the readings say its electrical vibration is altered by the other ingredients so that it will help relieve the pain without having the negative effect a narcotic alone, or a hypnotic will usually have on the body.

CATARACTS

Overview

1. Occur when the crystalline lens of the eye becomes increasingly clouded or opaque.

2. Result in a progressive, painless loss of vision; cataracts are the most common cause of blindness in the U.S.

3. There are many kinds of cataracts; the two main categories are developmental and degenerative cataracts.

Causes

1. Lens protein is believed to denature and to recoagulate, forming opaque areas; the readings refer to this as the formation of a chrysalis (or cocoon); later, calcium, insoluble sugars, and other molecules can be trapped inside this webbing, further worsening the situation.

2. This process can be initially started by poor ocular circulation, spinal lesions, and improper nerve impulses; the initial trigger for this could be an injury to the eye itself (either as trauma or from other causes), infection, other inflammatory processes, certain systemic diseases, certain medications, and debilitation in general.

Treatment

1. The Cayce readings indicate that the accumulations could be reabsorbed, but the process would be a slow one.

2. Osteopathic adjustments, especially in the upper cervicals and upper dorsals, to both help stimulate the circulation and improve the eliminations as the "cysts" were broken up.

3. Follow the "normal diet" as outlined in Chapter Seven, with a special emphasis on B vitamin supplements, seafood, and carrots or carrot juice.

4. Maintain a positive, constructive attitude.

5. Use the violet-ray applicator directly over the eyes (with them closed) to break up the accumulations and over the posterior neck to "enliven" the nerve centers.

6. General massage to help improve eliminations, most often with peanut oil; occasionally special attention to the face, head, and neck region is indicated.

7. As usual, therapies are to be done in cycles.

8. Use the head and neck exercises.

9. Apply Glyco-Thymoline packs to the eyes to help prevent further accumulations.

10. Use poultices of grated potatoes applied to the eyes for 30 minutes at a time; this is to help draw out some of the assorted accumulations.

11. The violet-ray applications and potato poultices are to followed by an eyewash of cleansing or boric acid solutions.

12. Eliminations are to be maintained with either laxatives, enemas, or colonics.

13. Fume baths with witch hazel or pine oil.

CEREBRAL PALSY

Overview

1. Any disorder of movement and/or posture that results from non-progressive damage to a developing brain.

2. May be associated with epilepsy, varying degrees of mental retardation, and speech and hearing difficulties.

Causes

1. Controversy currently exists over whether the damage to the nervous system occurs at birth, before birth, or some combination of the two; in the eighteen cases in the readings, 50 percent were stated to be birth-related, 22 percent were prenatal in origin, 6 percent were postnatal, and for 22 percent the origin of the damage was not specified.
2. Is often stated as being a karmic condition, both for the involved soul and for those close to him or her.
3. In addition to nerve damage, the Cayce readings indicate the condition often involved an incoordination of the three nervous systems, especially in the areas of "greater coordination"—most often given as the first through fourth cervical, the second through fourth dorsal, the ninth dorsal, and the second through fourth lumbar.
4. The lacteal ducts are also occasionally seen as not working properly, producing an impoverished blood and lymph supply of nutrients needed by the nerves.

Treatment

1. The earlier in life the treatments are begun the better, as after the "third cycle" (21 years of age) the condition might "become encased."
2. Are aimed at regenerating the nervous system, the readings repeatedly state this was possible but often required 7 to 10 years of consistent therapy; recent statistics show that in "mild cases" of cerebral palsy, 35 to 86 percent have complete resolution of symptoms by their seventh birthday.
3. It is emphasized that the treatment needs to be not only at the physical level but at the spiritual and mental levels as well; this will involve prayer, keeping a positive mental attitude, and the living of spiritual lives by those involved in the therapy.
4. The therapy, insofar as possible, is to be carried out by those close to the involved soul (such as the parents), as the condition in-

cludes lessons for them also, and is to be given with care, patience, and kindness.

5. To regenerate the nerves, the wet cell is used in a variety of ways; two of the more common ways are using gold chloride alone daily or alternating the gold chloride and Atomidine (connections for the gold are positive (+) at the ninth dorsal or fourth lumbar and negative (–) at the umbilical/lacteal center; for the Atomidine positive (+) at the second or fourth dorsal and negative (-) at the umbilical/lacteal center).

6. The wet-cell treatment is to be followed by gentle circular massage over the spine, paying especially close attention to the second through fourth cervical, second and third dorsal, ninth dorsal, and fourth lumbar using an olive oil/myrrh combination or cocoa butter in younger children; occasionally, it is recommended that the massage is to proceed down the legs, paying special attention to the feet.

7. One to two times a month, deeper treatments such as osteopathic adjustments are to be had in place of the massage.

CORONARY HEART DISEASE

Overview

1. The two major manifestations of coronary heart disease are myocardial infarctions (heart attacks) and angina pectoris; the underlying problem in both is that the heart's oxygen supply will not keep up with the oxygen demand.

2. It is the leading cause of mortality and morbidity in the industrialized world—causing a third of all deaths in the U.S.

3. It has been linked with a number of risk factors, the five primary ones being (a) elevated serum cholesterol, (b) high blood pressure, (c) smoking, (d) diabetes, and (e) a strong family history of the disease.

Causes

1. Ninety-five percent of all coronary heart disease is due to atherosclerotic plaques—calcified, ulcerated and fibrotic fat deposits in the arteries.

2. The exact cause of these plaques is still unknown by traditional medicine—they are, however, the culmination of a slow process which begins in early childhood.

3. The Cayce readings propose that the plaques result from a combination of poor eliminations, an unbalanced circulation, and excessive fat in the diet; three conditions that can contribute to produce this condition were given as a prolapsed or engorged colon, spinal lesions, and a congested liver.

4. These factors interact as follows:

    a. First, an improper diet and poor assimilation produce poisons in the system.

    b. Second, the colon and occasionally the liver do not adequately deal with these toxins.

    c. And finally, spinal lesions and the engorged colon create an unbalanced circulation (which can manifest as high blood pressure), which contributes to plaque formation and in the later stages of the disease place a direct burden on the heart.

Treatment

1. Eliminate red meat, fried foods, and fats from the diet; all of these contribute to an increased serum cholesterol and worsen the all-important HDL/LDL ratio; research has shown that for each 1 percent drop in serum cholesterol there is a 2 to 3 percent drop in the risk of a heart attack; also as serum cholesterol is lowered, the process of plaque formation can actually reverse.

2. Osteopathic manipulations are highly recommended as well; emphasis should be placed on the mid-dorsals to affect the circulatory balance between the heart, liver, and lungs directly and on

lumbosacral lesions which will enhance the functioning of the colon; some professional judgement needs to be exercised here— the readings indicate that the further along the symptoms have progressed, the gentler the treatments should become, moving more to a massage mode; also, care in these cases should be exercised in the dorsal region as stimulation of the sympathetic nervous system in some cases would be inadvisable.

3. Colonic irrigations are recommended to improve the eliminations of "poisons" and thus relieve the strain on the heart; these are to be given "professionally and scientifically" with great care to ensure a strain is not placed on the heart (this is to be gauged by monitoring the pulse); to be given in a series spaced 10 days apart until all the mucus is gone from the rinse waters—this goal is to be accomplished gradually and not attempted in just one or two treatments; the water is to be at body temperature with a level tablespoon of salt and a level teaspoon of soda added to each gallon of water; the final rinse waters are to contain Glyco-Thymoline.

4. If chest pain is experienced, physical and mental rest is mandated.

5. The impedance device is occasionally recommended as a way to help balance the circulation.

6. Medications are to be used as necessary to help acutely, but over time, as conditions improve, are to be discontinued.

DYSMENNORHEA (PAINFUL MENSTRUATION)

Overview

1. Onset of primary dysmennorhea is usually in adolescence, within 2 years of menarche.

2. Characterized by painful menstrual cramping, it can also be associated with diarrhea, vomiting, headaches, dizziness, irritability, and difficulty with concentration.

Causes

1. Believed to be caused by an excess of prostaglandins, which form naturally as part of the menstrual cycle in response to the hormone progesterone; these cause excessive contractions of the uterus, depriving it of oxygen and producing the pain.

2. From the Cayce readings' perspective, the cause of this buildup is an improper blood circulation through the uterus, hampering eliminations and causing an increased acidity.

3. The three most common causes of this impaired circulation are "spinal lesions" (see Chapter Six), a "tilted uterus," and "cold or congestion" in the pelvic region as the result of a viral illness.

Treatment

1. Heated sea-salt packs applied to the pubic area to help with the relief of pain; occasionally, this is alkalinized with the addition of Glyco-Thymoline or sodium bicarbonate.

2. Osteopathic adjustments with special attention to the lumbar and sacral regions of the spine.

3. Follow the diet outlined in Chapter Seven.

4. To help reduce local acidity and assist local glandular funtioning, douches are recommended for use in between periods; they are to be used every other day—alternating Atomidine and Glyco-Thymoline, one for a month and then the other the following month (both are to be mixed in the ratio of 1 teaspoon to 1 quart of warm water).

5. Violet-ray applications over the lower back.

6. General massages.

7. Take time to rest, both physically and mentally, while the symptoms are occurring.

EPILEPSY

Overview

1. A term applied to group of disorders, characterized by episodes in which abnormal electrical discharges in the brain spread and cause "electrical storms," resulting in seizures.

2. Can be divided into a primary disorder—where seizures are the only problem—and a secondary disorder—where the epileptic attacks are associated with a known problem with the nervous system such as scarring following a stroke, surgery, or other trauma; the causes and treatments outlined here relate to the primary form of epilepsy.

3. Seizures, though intermittent, are evidence of continual abnormal interactions between portions of the nervous system which persist between epileptic attacks; this can be measured as brief, high-amplitude electrical discharges with the use of an EEG.

Causes

1. Traditional medicine postulates that some form of cerebral lesion combines with a genetic predisposition to produce epilepsy.

2. The readings, in discussing primary epilepsy (the 50 percent of cases where a specific neural cause for the seizures cannot be found), concentrate on two types of lesions—lacteal duct lesions and spinal lesions.

3. Lacteal ducts are parts of the abdominal lymphatics involved in the absorption of fats from the gut; lesions in this area are said to interface with the flow of chyle through an actual constriction or narrowing of the lacteal vessels or from some type of spasming; the readings indicate that this could be detected at times as an actual cold spot in the right upper quadrant of the abdomen.

4. Lacteal duct lesions are often caused by a reflex reaction from an injury to the spinal column—most commonly in the sacral/coccyxgeal region; direct trauma to the right upper quadrant of the

abdomen or to the umbilical region during the birth process are also given as causes.

5. These lacteal duct lesions have far-reaching effects via the autonomic nervous system, and could affect eliminations, alter hepatic circulation, interfere with oxidative processes in the body, and produce spinal lesions—most commonly in the sacral/coccyxgeal region, ninth and tenth dorsals, and the first through third cervicals.

6. The spinal and lacteal duct lesions can combine to produce an incoordination between the central and autonomic nervous systems.

7. Autonomic nervous system reflexive activity also affects the endocrine system—specifically, the adrenals and gonads—which then can trigger responses in the pineal and pituitary glands.

8. The end result of this incoordination is an imbalance of nerve centers in the brain stem (in the medulla oblongata), leading to an overflow of neuronal discharge, which spreads to the cortex and produces a seizure.

Treatment

1. Traditional medicine uses drugs that sedate the nerves and slow their rate of firing; the readings focus on dealing with the lacteal duct and spinal lesions which they cite as the cause of the problem.

2. Hot castor oil packs are recommended to break up the lesions and adhesions in the lacteal duct area; these are usually placed over the entire right side of the abdomen for 1 to 3 hours at a time and given in 3-day series.

3. To help break up the lacteal duct lesions, the abdomen should be kneaded and massaged immediately after the castor oil pack; peanut oil or olive oil and myrrh or all three together are recommended as the massage oil.

4. Olive oil (usually 2 tablespoons) is to be taken at bedtime on the last day of the pack series to nourish the cells of the lacteal ducts.

5. Osteopathic massage and manipulation are to *follow* each series of castor oil packs to influence the balance between the autonomic and central nervous systems; correcting this imbalance will also help restore proper functioning of the endocrine system.

6. Diet is to be watched closely and the general Cayce diet, outlined in Chapter Seven, is recommended.

7. Gastrointestinal eliminations are to be maintained with the use of laxatives or colonics.

8. A boiled concentrate from the passion flower (also known as the maypop or mayflower) is recommended to replace the use of other sedatives; taking 1 teaspoonful four times a day, it is supposed to have a calming effect on the nervous system; the readings occasionally approve the temporary continuation of Dilantin and Phenobarbital; the goal, however, is the eventual elimination of the need to use these types of drugs.

HYPOTHYROIDISM

Overview

1. A clinical syndrome which results from a deficiency of thyroid hormone; common symptoms include weakness and fatigue, dry and coarse skin, cold intolerance and decreased sweating, weight gain despite a decreased appetite, constipation, muscle cramps, and impaired hearing.

2. Generally, affects women (in a 14:1 ratio to men) over the age of forty, but can occur at any age.

3. Many of the cases in the readings probably represent a "sluggish" thyroid as opposed to the full-blown clinical syndrome.

Causes

1. The two major causes of hypothyroidism are (a) an apparent autoimmune destruction of the thyroid gland, and (b) thyroid destruction resulting from radiation or surgical treatment for

hyperthyroidism; the material in the readings applies mainly to the first category.

2. The Cayce readings indicate that hypothyroidism is primarily a glandular problem, most often resulting from a lack of certain elements in the bloodstream combined with the accumulation of "poisons" from poor eliminations.

3. Other factors can contribute to this situation, including spinal lesions, an increase in body acidity, worry, and a decrease in stimulation to the thyroid gland from the sympathetic nervous system; the lacteal ducts and adrenal glands also seem to play a role in this process.

4. The results of this interplay include an unbalancing of the ratio of iodides to potashes (potassium), which further aggravates the condition; calcium also appears to be important in this process.

5. Hypothyroidism also effects the balance of the superficial and deep circulation, the hepatic circulation, other endocrine glands, and the kidneys.

Treatment

1. Therapy is directed at stimulating and cleansing the glandular system, assisting proper assimilation, and stimulating the superficial circulation.

2. The cyclic use of Atomidine is recommended to both stimulate and balance glandular function.

3. General osteopathic adjustments and gentle massage using olive oil and myrrh are suggested to help balance both the nervous systems and the circulation.

4. Other measures recommended to help rebalance the circulatory patterns include the use of an impedance device, alternating hot and cold packs, and sweat baths followed by a rubdown.

5. Dietary suggestions center on the intake of a more alkaline diet and the assimilation of certain elements—including iron, silicon, calcium, phosphorus, and the iodides; foods that are especially

recommended include potato skins, orange juice, dried milks, and organ meats (such as liver and tripe).

6. Cod liver oil is recommended as a supplement when symptoms are very mild.

7. In cases where the hypothyroidism is fairly well progressed, the readings recommend the use of thyroid extract (thyroxine); one individual who was already taking this on the instructions of their doctor was told to continue to do so.

MULTIPLE SCLEROSIS

Overview

1. Characterized, as the name implies, by multiple areas within the nervous system of "sclerosed" or hardened tissue in which the cells insulating the nerve tracts are destroyed and replaced by scar tissue.

2. These areas distort or block the flow of messages in the nervous system and can produce a myriad of symptoms—ranging from visual problems to weakness and numbness to loss of bladder function.

3. Symptoms usually appear between the ages of twenty and forty; slightly more women than men develop multiple sclerosis (MS).

Causes

1. Despite 150 years of investigation, traditional medicine does not understand the etiology of MS; it is noted to occur more frequently in the northern latitudes with fewer cases noted near the equator—because of this, an environmental agent has been postulated; traditional medicine has strongly considered an infectious agent as this environmental cause but despite intensive searching, this agent has not been found; the readings explicitly deny that an infectious agent is responsible for MS (interestingly, there are more MS cases in areas with high standards of sanitation).

2. The readings cite a disequilibrium of the normal balance of metals in the body, produced primarily by a lack of gold in the system—this apparently combines with the liver not manufacturing enough of a certain substance and produces a glandular disturbance; the result is a hormonal imbalance which affects the nerves and their associated cells in the nervous system (so the readings might postulate the environmental factor to be the availability of gold).

3. This gold deficiency is tied to problems with its assimilation, which in turn is dependent on proper glandular functioning; in other words, there is a circular feedback relationship between gold, the involved glands, and the assimilation of gold.

4. While the affected hormone is not named, it is stated to be a nutrient to the nerve tissue; without this, a toxin can form in the nerve cells which causes the surrounding support cells to be poisoned and die—causing the sclerosing or hardening of the tissue around nerve cells which is associated with MS.

Treatment

1. The main objective is to awaken the body to the need for more gold. This is done with the use of the wet-cell battery. The use of gold in the solution jar is occasionally alternated with iodine (to stimulate the glands) or spirits of camphor (to help the functioning of the digestive system); as described in Chapter Ten, the negative (−) plate is placed over the umbilical and lacteal duct center in the right upper quadrant of the abdomen, and the positive (+) plate is placed at various locations along the spine—but most frequently over the ninth or tenth dorsal or the fourth lumbar area.

2. Iodine, to stimulate the glands (as mentioned above), is often recommended in one of several forms: iodine could be used in the solution jar, the wet cell could be "charged" with iodine, it could be taken orally in the form of Atomidine, or the quantity of dietary sources of iodine such as seafood could be increased.

3. A thorough massage of the spine and extremities is to follow the use of the wet cell; most commonly, a peanut oil/olive oil/lanolin mixture is to be used for this; the massage is usually to proceed from the spine out to the distal portions of the extremities using a circular motion.

4. Dietary recommendations are the same as those outlined in Chapter Seven, with an emphasis on foods which naturally carry large quantities of the B vitamins.

5. Treatment is stated to require time, with the above applications usually requiring 3 to 7 years to see full results.

PEPTIC ULCER DISEASE

Overview

1. Ulcers are defects in the mucosal lining of the digestive system, most often occurring either in the stomach or in the first portion of the small bowel known as the duodenum.

2. They are common, occurring in a fourth of all men and a sixth of all women in the U.S. and producing symptoms in 5 to 10 percent of the population.

Causes

1. The integrity of the cells lining the stomach and the small bowel depend on the production of a layer of mucus and bicarbonate, adequate blood flow, and cell renewal for protection.

2. Potentially damaging factors to these cells include acid, bile, and digestive enzymes from the stomach and the pancreas; these are controlled by nerve stimulation, pH, and the presence of food (especially protein and calcium) in the gut.

3. Ulcers occur when the balance between protectors of the cell lining and potentially damaging factors, both listed above, is upset.

4. From the Cayce readings' perspective, this imbalance can be caused by a number of factors, either acting singly or more commonly in a complex interplay with each other; these include:

    a. Emotional and/or physical overtaxation.

    b. A spinal lesion (most often in the dorsal area) causing improper nerve stimulation (either too little or too much) to the digestive organs and secretory cells.

    c. An impoverished or impaired blood flow, affecting the mucosal lining directly as well as causing the liver or pancreas to behave sluggishly.

    d. An overacidity of the entire system.

    e. Poor eliminations.

    f. An actual positioning problem of the stomach impairing the proper flow of digestive contents.

    g. Occasionally, the mucosal integrity was initially disrupted by a "flu-like" process or from the action of a medication.

5. According to the readings, these same factors would often produce other symptoms including changes in the sensory system (such as the eyes, ears, and taste), decreased vitality, headaches, anemia, and skin changes ranging from acne to boils.

Treatment

1. Traditional therapy focuses on decreasing the production of acid with H-2 blockers, neutralizing the acid with antacids, or shoring up the mucosal defenses with agents that coat the gut.

2. The readings' approach is twofold—first, correct as many of the causes listed above as possible, and second, take the necessary steps to protect and balance the stomach and intestinal mucosa.

3. To help accomplish these objectives, the following suggestions are given:

    a. All water consumed should either contain a pinch of elm bark or be yellow saffron tea; the elm bark is stated to help stabilize the mucus coating and also add to the alkaline reaction from the salivary glands, the saffron tea helps by buffering the pH—preventing both overacidity and overalkalinity—and also by giving a protective coating to the stomach, especially before a meal.

    b. The diet itself should consist of easily digested foods (arrowroot and junket are both specified) and little to no meat (though beef juice is allowed); both of these will result in faster passage through the stomach and decreased acid production.

c. Osteopathic adjustments, most commonly concentrating on the dorsal spine, to help balance nerve input; this requires a skilled practioner who can discern when and where to "stimulate" vs. "relax" the tissue.

d. Improve eliminations with a colonic or enema to help rid the body of poisons and increase general resistance and decrease the risk of the ulcer becoming malignant (in the case of gastric ulcers only); movement of bowel contents can also be helped with the use of moderate exercise, junket, and a mild bowel stimulant.

e. Improve vitality in general with the use of a radium appliance, ultraviolet rays, and/or carbonated ash.

f. Provide nutrients for the bowel mucosa with the occasional intake of olive oil.

4. The readings told several individuals that if they followed these suggestions for 6 months they would be able to "eat nails" if they desired without it adversely affecting their system.

PSORIASIS

Overview

1. A common chronic disorder which affects more than 1 million Americans.

2. Its major manifestations are red, dry, scaly plaques most commonly found over the knees, elbows, and scalp; it can also cause pitting of the nails and a form of arthritic joint pain.

3. It can begin at any age and its severity, course, and remissions are unpredictable.

Causes

1. The Cayce readings implicate the lack of proper coordination of the elimination systems causing a thinning of the walls of the

small intestine—specifically, the jejunum and the lower duo-denum—in the etiology of psoriasis.

2. This thinning allows toxic products to leak from the intestinal tract into the circulation; these eventually find their way into the superficial circulation and lymphatics and are eliminated through the skin, producing the plaques of psoriasis.

Treatment

1. Correct diet is emphasized; most commonly mentioned are one meal a day of fresh raw vegetables, the restriction of fats, starches, and sweets, no fried foods, the use of whole wheat products, and abstaining from eating red meats.

2. Yellow saffron tea and the use of powdered slippery elm in all drinking water are recommended for the healing of the intestinal walls; alternating mullein or chamomile tea with the yellow saffron tea is occasionally recommended.

3. Osteopathic manipulations, focusing on the mid-dorsals, to improve blood and lymph circulation in the abdomen are recommended.

4. Colonics are occasionally recommended to maintain proper eliminations patterns from the gut.

5. Most attention is focused on treating the underlying cause as opposed to the skin condition itself; however, plantain salve and camphorated oil are the most commonly mentioned of several topical applications to be used on the plaques.

RHEUMATOID ARTHRITIS

Overview

1. A chronic inflammatory disorder which primarily affects the small joints of the hands in a symmetrical fashion; it is characterized by swollen and painful joints and morning stiffness.

2. Can also affect many other joints including the elbows, wrists, shoulders, knees, feet, and ankles; it can also affect a number of organ systems in the body.

3. Women are affected two to three times more often than men and the peak incidence is between the fourth and sixth decades of life.

4. The onset is usually insidious, taking weeks to months; it often starts with fatigue, malaise and diffuse aches and pains; it has a highly variable clinical course ranging from a mild disease of brief duration to a progressive, destructive, and crippling arthritis.

Causes

1. The etiology remains elusive to researchers despite intensive investigation; the two most promising lines of thought involve (a) some form of abnormality of the immune system and its regulation, and (b) a search for an infectious agent.

2. The Cayce readings propose that a number of factors, acting in concert, play a role in the etiology of rheumatoid arthritis; most commonly mentioned is a glandular disturbance which alters the individual's assimilation of nutrients—this could lead to actual deficiencies in the blood levels of certain elements.

3. Eliminations are also often disturbed and toxins are left in the lymph and blood stream; specifically, an incoordination between the liver and kidneys is given as causing the poor elimination pattern.

Treatment

1. Traditionally, since the cause of rheumatoid arthritis is unknown, therapy has focused on relief of pain and reduction of the inflammation.

2. The diet, according to the Cayce readings, should contain lots of carrots, watercress, celery, and lettuce; raw vegetables, in general, should become a greater portion of the food consumed.

3. Iodine, in one form or another, is recommended to help correct the glandular dysfunction; half the time, this involves using the wet-cell battery "charged with iodine"; another option is to use Atomidine taken orally.

4. Another element recommended to help rejuvenate the body's glands was gold; the wet-cell battery is most commonly recommended to deliver this influence to the body; interestingly, gold is one of the few forms of treatment in traditional medicine which is felt to occasionally lead to a "cure" of rheumatoid arthritis; gold, however, is often poorly tolerated with many side effects when taken directly—the wet cell, in theory, allows the body to access gold more naturally (see Chapter Ten).

5. Epsom salts are recommended to help break up the collection of toxins at the involved joints; this usually takes the form of a hot Epsom-salt bath; in cases where a hot bath might not be well tolerated, Epsom salt packs are to be placed over the affected joint.

6. Massage is also universally recommended; the timing of the massage is important—it is to be given during or immediately following the epsom-salt bath; similarly, if the wet-cell battery is used, it is to be followed by a massage; when massage is given separately from the bath, either peanut oil by itself or combined with olive and pine needle oil is recommended.

7. The readings often warn individuals that they would initially get worse with these treatments before they got better; if the therapy was not going to be followed consistently and persistently, it would be better not to start the process at all.

SCHIZOPHRENIA

Overview

1. A devastating disturbance of mind and personality which can include auditory hallucinations, delusions, and altered behavior toward others.

2. The most common psychotic disorder—it affects over 2 million Americans and 1 percent of people worldwide.

3. Most schizophrenics are psychotic for only a small part of their lives—in between episodes the individuals may be withdrawn, isolated, and "peculiar."

Causes

1. No consistent structural or functional abnormality has been found in schizophrenics to give a clue as to its origins; it is felt to be the result of a genetic predisposition combined with influences from the individual's social and family interactions, often initiated by some form of adversity.

2. The Cayce readings refer to hereditary and/or karmic influences and the effects of negative emotions, but most commonly, they refer to spinal injuries or pressures as the beginning of the process which becomes schizophrenia.

3. These spinal lesions, usually in the lower spine and most commonly involving the coccyx, produce incoordination of the central and the sympathetic nervous systems; this incoordination can be seen in the early signs of a relapse which include restlessness and nervousness, loss of appetite, mild depression, insomnia, and trouble concentrating.

4. These pressures also affect the functioning of glands which are specifically mentioned elsewhere in the readings as the regulators of our spiritual energy—the gonads, cells of Leydig, and the pineal gland.

5. As these centers are affected, if there was a concommitant failure to engage in spiritual service arising from an ideal, then mental aberrations would slowly occur and the functioning of the nervous system, over time, would become progressively depleted and distorted.

Treatment

1. Traditionally, treatment now rests on a combination of pharmaceutical and psychosocial methods; the Cayce readings combine physical and social interventions as well.

2. Osteopathic manipulations are recommended to correct the spinal lesions with an emphasis on the coccyx, sacral, and lumbar spine.

3. Use of the wet-cell battery with gold chloride is suggested to rejuvenate the nervous system and improve glandular functioning; the impedance device is also recommended to help coordinate the different components of the nervous system to work together better.

4. Massage is recommended to help relax the individual and coordinate the nervous systems as well.

5. A complete change of environment, taking the individual out of their current situation, is also suggested; chronic hospitalization has been shown to have deleterious effects and studies have also shown that a return "home" after hospitalization produces a faster relapse.

6. Provide the individual with a constant companion who is close in age to them; this companion is to treat the individual with kindness, persistence, prayer, love, and gentleness.

7. Use positive suggestions, including nightly presleep suggestions, to help direct the individual's behavior.

8. Follow closely the dietary recommendations made in Chapter Seven.

9. Engage in outdoor activity, exercise, and physical work involving the hands.

APPENDIX A

Answers to Common Questions and Remedies for Common Complaints

Q: *Did the readings have anything to say about the acquired immune deficiency syndrome (AIDS)?*

A: No. The last Cayce reading was given in 1944 and so they do not directly address any cases of AIDS. However, we can conjecture what their approach might have been. AIDS is now known to be caused by a virus, which has been called the human immunodeficiency virus (HIV). Three principal directions have been taken in seeking a cure: to produce a vaccine against the virus, to identify drugs which kill the virus, and to identify therapies which enhance the immune system. It can *safely* be said that the Cayce readings would have sided with the third approach.

First, the person with AIDS should attempt a general strengthening of the body following the health principles outlined in Part One of this book. This regimen involves examining and working with mental and spiritual patterns, improving diet, beginning a regular nonstrenuous exercise program, working with techniques to relax the body, coordinating the nervous systems with the use of spinal adjustments, and helping the four organs of elimination to work optimally. If nothing more, this should help reduce the number of secondary infections a person experiences, thereby slowing the disease process.

In addition, a number of specific steps to help the immune system might be extrapolated from the readings. Each would be aimed at helping the depleted T-helper cells rejuvenate themselves. These include:

- Proper attitude, making sure not to overtax the body with mental or physical strain.

- The daily consumption of carrots, lettuce, and celery. The readings indicate this helps "insure against any contagious infectious forces" (no. 480–19). Lettuce is also said to supply an "effluvium in the blood stream itself that is a destructive force to *most* of those influences that attack the blood stream" (no. 404–6).
- The use of the wet-cell battery with gold chloride. This is said to stimulate "an increase in the numbers of the leucocyte that are the warriors" (no. 988–7). The use of gold chloride with the wet cell is also said to be helpful in "rejuvenating any organ of the system showing the delinquency in action" (no. 1800–6). This would be used every 2 to 3 days.
- The use of cyclic doses of Atomidine (iodine trichloride). The readings state that Atomidine "will purify the glandular system so as to resist adverse influences" (no. 1521–2). A standard regimen would be to start with 1 drop of Atomidine in a half a glass of water first thing in the morning. The next morning 2 drops would be used; the third morning, 3 drops. The fourth and fifth days would then taper the dosage; 2 drops the fourth day, 1 drop the fifth day. This cycle of 5 days would be repeated every 28 days.
- The use of beef juice to help with "strength and vitality." (Directions for making this are on page 189.) This is to be taken a teaspoonful at a time, four times a day, and sipped slowly.
- Plantain salve is recommended for skin lesions, including cancer, and may be helpful with Kaposi's sarcoma.
- To help activate the immune cells in the lungs, as in cases of tuberculosis, the readings recommend the use of a charred oak keg. This is to be filled with 100-proof apple brandy and the fumes inhaled. This may prove helpful with some of the atypical pulmonary infections associated with AIDS.

Q: *What do the readings say about smoking?*

A: Many people are perplexed when they discover that Edgar Cayce was a chain smoker and that the readings say that smoking in moderation is okay. It's important to place this in perspective. The readings state that moderation means three to six cigarettes a day, which statistically does not place an individual at increased risk of lung cancer. Of course, it is rare to find an individual who exhibits such moderation. The readings Cayce gave for himself were direct in telling him that he should reduce his smoking because it was harming him. The readings tell some individuals to never start smoking because it would be habit-forming for them (25 to 28 percent of smokers are addicted to the nicotine in cigarette smoke) and any addiction is harmful.

Times have changed since the readings were given. The readings recommend "natural leaf" as having less harmful potential, but such tobacco is now hard to come by. Cigarettes today have numerous harmful chemicals—added during processing—which are known to be carcinogenic. Because of these chemicals and the process of pyrosynthesis which occurs at the cigarette tip, the smoke is now thought to be more damaging to people near smokers than to the smokers themselves. In addition, smoking—in today's society—carries with it connotations of being inconsiderate, feelings of guilt, and the expectancy of eventual disease. Because of these changes, smoking cigarettes is no longer compatible with a healthful lifestyle.

Q: *How do the readings approach the common cold?*

A: The Cayce readings emphasize that the statement that each of our bodies is "a law unto itself" is especially true when considering the common cold. Because of this, they call the cold "one of the most erratic conditions that may be considered as an ill to the human body" (no. 902–1). Acknowledging that colds are caused by a contagious germ that attacks the mucous membrances, the readings stress the role of prevention.

The body's acid-base balance plays an important role in this prevention. An excess in either direction, but most commonly involving an excessive acidic-state, causes an individual to become more susceptible. The readings indicate that the cold germ reproduces more easily when the body is in acidic-state and finds it difficult to live in an alkaline state. When we are physically depleted, for any reason, our bodies tend to be in an acidic state and hence more likely to catch a cold.

During these times, changes in temperature, drafts, and getting the feet damp can all affect the body's circulatory balance and further increase susceptibility. The readings indicate that even a heightened psychological awareness that the appropriate environmental conditions exist makes it easier to catch a cold.

As a result, precautions should be taken when such a predisposition exists. These would include:

- The short-term use of a vitamin supplement at those times when the body is susceptible. The readings indicate that an abundant supply of *all* vitamins is helpful.
- The maintenance of a balanced diet, protecting against foods that produce an excess of acidity—especially sweets.
- Wearing appropriate clothing for the environmental conditions and protecting against drafts and dampness.
- Keeping rested.

Once a cold has attacked a body, the readings indicate that certain measures should always be taken:

- Rest! The cold itself indicates "exhaustion" somewhere in the body. Additionally, the inflamation of the mucous membrances itself weakens the body and rest helps protect any other weakened portions of the system from being affected.
- Determine the body's initial weak link and work to restore balance in this area. Most commonly, the problem is a lack of proper eliminations. In this case, drinking increased quantities of water and the use of an alkalinizer such as citrus juice or a teaspoon of baking soda to a glass of water sipped slowly every hour is helpful. The diet should consist of foods that are easily assimilated and for this reason be mainly liquids. Heavy foods such as meats and fried foods should be avoided.

Q: *What are some of the remedies suggested by the readings to help with the congestion and coughing that can accompany an upper respiratory infection?*

A: To help with congestion, the readings recommend several options:

- The most common suggestion for congestion and sinus problems is the use of an inhalant. Different formulas are given, but in general, an alcohol inhalant is recommended for the upper respiratory tract and a steam inhalant for the lower respiratory tract. Common formulas for these are:

Ingredients	Steam Inhalant	Alcohol Inhalant
Grain alcohol	none	4 ounces
Oil of eucalyptus	180 milliliters	30 minims
Oil of turpentine	60 milliliters	10 minims
Oil of pine needles	10 milliliters	5 minims
Balsam of tolu	10 milliliters	15 minims
Compound tincture of benzoin	240 milliliters	20 minims

(1 milliliter = approximately 15 minums; 1 minim = approximately 1 drop)

- Another option is to massage a compound made from equal parts of mutton tallow, spirits of turpentine, and spirits of camphor—twice a day—into the feet, legs, and ankles, and also on the chest and throat. To make the compound, warm and strain the mutton tallow and then add the other ingredients.
- Finally, one can use a Glyco-Thymoline (a treatment for mucosity and a mouthwash) pack: this is made by soaking two to three thicknesses

of cotton cloth with prewarmed Glyco-Thymoline. This is placed directly over the nares and sinus areas for 15 to 20 minutes.

For coughs, the readings gave a number of formulas using syrup of wild cherry bark and syrup of horehound as active ingredients. The addition of glycerine is often recommended to soothe the throat. One individual was given the following formula, which might be easier to make in the home setting:

"For any flu or cold, *this* would be well as an expectorant and as an eliminant, and to cause the clearing of hoarseness—made in this way and manner:

"Take an egg that has *not* been in the refrigerator or cold storage. Take the white of same. Beat it.

"Then, to this white of egg, add:

"Juice of one lemon, dropped very slowly into same. About a teaspoonful of honey, dropped slowly into same also. About *three* drops—one at a time—of glycerine.

"Beat thoroughly together. Of course, it would be worked in together when the glycerine is added.

"Take a teaspoonful every 2 or 3 hours.

"We will find this will clear a cold, relieve stress through the throat and the nasal passages, bronchi and larynx, and be most helpful for this body" (no. 845–3).

Q: *Are there any suggestions for maintaining the health of the eyes?*

A: General recommendations include maintaining the cervical and upper dorsal vertebrae in proper alignment and consuming raw vegetables (especially carrots) with gelatin and citrus fruits as part of the diet. To specifically help maintain visual acuity, the readings recommend the daily use of the head-and-neck exercises, as described in Chapter Nine.

For tired and irritated eyes, the readings suggest bathing the eyes with a solution of one-third Glyco-Thymoline and two-thirds distilled water. Potato poultices are also suggested for irritated eyes and/or for inflammation of the eyelids. To make a poultice, use an *old* Irish potato and *scrape* the potato with a paring knife. This will produce a mushlike material which is placed directly on the closed eyelids and bound with a cloth for half an hour to an hour. The scraping breaks open the cells of the potato and apparently releases enzymes which help draw out the inflammation. After the potato poultice is removed, the eyes should be rinsed with a weak antiseptic cleansing solution, such as boric acid.

Q: *Did the readings discuss hemorrhoids?*

A: Hemorrhoids result from the distention of the network of veins located around the anus and rectum. The readings state that this can occur from a number of factors that range from prolapsus of the colon and other elimination problems that cause congestion in the alimentary canal to spinal injuries which affect the nerves in the sphincter area.

Therapy consists of a local topical application, a specific stretching exercise, increased dietary fiber, improved elimination patterns (which includes occasional colonics), and correction of spinal lesions.

The readings give the formula for a topical astringent, nicknamed "TIM," to help shrink the hemorrhoids. It is composed of iodine and benzoin in a base of butterfat and tobacco. It is the topical ointment most recommended by the readings for the treatment of hemorrhoids. For internal hemorrhoids, TIM can be heated and injected with a syringe. A combination of carbolic acid (also called phenol; still used for this purpose today), glycerine, and Nujol (an equivalent of Russian White Oil)is also recommended as an injection.

The recommended exercise is the morning setting-up exercise described in Chapter Nine. It improves muscle tone and helps decrease congestion by improving lymphatic and venous flow.

Q: *Did anyone receive advice on varicose veins?*

A: The readings explain that varicose veins originate from an impaired circulation and damage to the vessel wall. The condition can be produced by a combination of mechanical trauma, increased venous pressure, and a buildup of toxins in the slowed superficial circulation that may damage the vessels themselves. Spinal lesions in the lumbar and sacral areas can also contribute to a slowed circulation and to the actual dilatation of the blood vessels.

Therapy consists of correcting spinal lesions, massaging the affected limbs, and the use of elastic support hose to help venous return. The massage involves working from distal to proximal with the use of olive oil and myrrh (occasionally combined with tincture of benzoin) as the massage oil.

The readings also recommend the use of the mullein plant. The leaves can be used dry or fresh as a tea or fresh leaves can be made into a stupe which is placed directly on the varicose veins. The tea is said to help coordinate the circulation through the abdominal organs, thereby easing pressure in the lower extremities. The stupes are made by bruising mullein leaves, pouring boiling water over them, and applying them over the affected areas when they have cooled enough so that they don't burn.

Q: *What is the best way to care for the gums and teeth?*

A: In addition to the use of other toothpastes, the Cayce readings recommend the use of equal parts table salt (occasionally calcium chloride was used in place of sodium chloride) and baking soda for use as a dentifrice three to four times a week to help keep the teeth clean. To help prevent cavities, the readings suggest rinsing the mouth once a month, before brushing, with a pint of water in which a drop of chlorine has been added (this is NOT to be swallowed). The readings also suggest the use of a series of calcium supplements during the second year of each 7-year cycle, which is when the teeth undergo greater cyclic changes, according to the readings. Once cavities have developed, the readings recommend filling them with something other than heavy metals like gold.

Inflammation of the gums, such as gingivitis and the more serious condition of pyorrhea, is a very common condition in the United States. For these conditions, the readings recommend a preparation nicknamed "IPSAB." The principal ingredient is prickly ash bark, which the Indians called "toothache bark." To this, sea water, calcium chloride or sodium chloride, iodine trichloride (Atomidine) and essence of peppermint are added. In severe cases, this is massaged thoroughly into the gums for 5 minutes, twice a day, using one's finger. After the massage, the mouth is rinsed with undiluted Glyco-Thymoline or Lavoris followed by tap water. *Do not* swallow any of these solutions. These same combinations are recommended as treatments for canker sores as well. Another option is to dab the canker sore with Atomidine followed by a Glyco-Thymoline rinse.

Q: *What ideas do the readings have to help prevent or reduce obesity?*

A: The Cayce readings indicate that obesity results not only from "an excess of starches in the diet," but also from an interplay of other factors. These include poor elimination patterns and an incoordination of the nervous system which can combine to produce glandular imbalance. All of these lead to an altered metabolism of sugar.

The most common suggestion is a series of general osteopathic adjustments to help coordinate the nervous system and improve circulation and elimination patterns. Massage is also commonly recommended for similar reasons. Adipose tissue is known to be richly innervated by fibers of the autonomic nervous system and coordinating the nervous system may affect the neuronal messages going and coming from the fat cells themselves.

To improve elimination patterns, colonics and/or vapor baths are also suggested.

To help with appetite and correcting the altered sugar metabolism, the readings recommend the use of diluted Concord grape juice—two parts juice to one part water—to be taken half an hour before each meal and before retiring. The readings say this provides the body with a type of sugar which does not promote weight gain and will help rebalance the body's sugar metabolism. Fifty percent of the naturally occurring sugar in grape juice is fructose. Research has shown that a small dose of fructose before a meal decreases the amount of food consumed at the meal by 30 percent. Other effects that grape juice may have on the body still need further exploring.

Q: *Any suggestions for fractures, sprains, and other soft tissue swelling?*

A: For any healing fracture (once the cast is off) or sprain, the readings recommend the use of table salt moistened with pure apple cider vinegar as a rub or a pack. Often, this is to be applied as hot as the individual can tolerate. The readings indicate that this combination may produce discomfort at times but is therapeutically beneficial.

A formula in which Russian White Oil, witch hazel, tincture of benzoin, oil of sassafras, and kerosene are added to olive oil is said to help relieve the swelling and pain associated with sprains, strained muscles, and bruises.

Q: *What are some remedies to help with the care of the skin, nails, and hair?*

A: The following are an assortment of remedies for common problems with the skin, nails, and hair:

- *For scars:* A formula including camphorated olive oil, lanolin, and peanut oil is recommended; it is to be gently massaged into the scar tissue twice a day—with the process requiring 3 to 6 months for dissolution of the scar (camphorated olive oil is now very difficult to obtain).
- *For warts:* use equal portions of castor oil and baking soda to make a gumlike substance to massage over the wart; this can be covered with a band-aid; it may initially produce irritation before there is resolution of the condition.
- *For callouses:* Start by massaging the callous with baking soda which has been moistened with spirits of camphor; after 5 to 10 days, change to olive oil and tincture of myrrh as the massage oil.
- *For moles:* Massage with castor oil twice a day.
- *For ingrown nails:* Use either (1) a small amount of cotton saturated with Atomidine, or (2) baking soda moistened with castor oil and placed under the points or edges where the ingrown nail is irritating the skin; in the case of the baking soda and castor oil, this is to be rubbed off with spirits of camphor.

- *To strengthen nails:* Apply a paste made from pure apple cider vinegar and table salt to the nails or massage the cuticles with Atomidine (this may cause some coloring of the nail).
- *For poor hair condition or hair loss:* Consider the cyclic use of Atomidine or dietary sources of iodine such as potato skins and seafood to help stimulate the functioning of the thyroid gland. As a local application, the readings recommend the use of a crude oil massage to the scalp. The oil may be left for 30 to 45 minutes; then rinsed out with a 20 percent grain alcohol solution and finished by massaging a small amount of white petroleum jelly (Vaseline) into the scalp.
- *For dandruff:* Either (1) use Listerine at one shampoo and Lavoris at the next, or (2) take 4 ounces of pure water and add 1.5 cc's of 85 percent alcohol with 2 minims of oil of pine, massage thoroughly into the scalp, and, while the hair is still damp, massage a small quantity of Vaseline thoroughly into the scalp, then wash the hair thoroughly with a tar soap (this is to be done about once a week).

Q: *Did the readings ever give any foods a special healing connotation?*

A: Yes, the following are foods that qualify for such a distinction:

- *Almonds* are said to contain a type of vitamin that helps prevent cancer and skin blemishes. The readings suggest an almond a day as a preventative measure.
- *Jerusalem artichokes* (a plant with a tuberous root and a top like a sunflower) is recommended for diabetics and for people with a tendency to run high sugars. It apparently helps rebalance the pancreas, liver, and kidneys. Most commonly, the readings recommend that it be *steamed* in Patapar paper and eaten about once a week.
- *Gelatin* is said to have the ability to help the glands function better by giving them the ability to use the vitamins which are in the system. It is often recommended that raw vegetables and salads be eaten with gelatin added.
- *Beef juice* is recommended as an invigorator and for general strengthening of a debilatated or weakened body. It is not beef broth, but a juice extracted from meat through the process of heat. (The meat is placed in a glass jar which sits for 3 to 4 hours in simmering water. The juice is to be taken a teaspoonful at a time, 4 times a day.)
- *Mummy food* is described as "almost a spiritual food for the body." The name came from a dream of Edgar Cayce's in which a mummy came to life and gave the recipe to Cayce. (It is made by cooking 1 cup of chopped black figs, 1 cup of chopped dates, ¼ cup of yellow cornmeal, and 2 to 3 cups of water over low heat for 10 to 15 minutes. It can be served with milk or cream.)

APPENDIX B

The Cayce Health Readings: A Historical Perspective

An editorial, "Holistic Health or Hoax?", appeared in the March 1979 *Journal of the American Medical Association*. It stated, in part, that "the roots of present-day holism probably go back 100 years to the birth of Edgar Cayce in Hopkinsville, Kentucky." While flattering, the statement suggests either an ignorance or a denial of the history of medicine. It also, in my opinion, lumps the Cayce health readings with a group of largely ignored philosophies and, as a result, prevents the serious researcher from examining them.

During his lifetime Edgar Cayce gave more than nine thousand "physical readings" for more than six thousand individuals. This productivity translates into a massive amount of information and also raises legitimate questions: Of what significance is all this information? Are these thousands of readings merely the legacy of a well-known psychic or do they contain information of actual value? Likewise, if the roots of holistic medicine predate Cayce, what role might the readings play in the return of biology to a spiritual perspective?

A brief look at the history of medicine provides some fascinating answers to these questions.

Historically, there have been two major ways to approach the human body and the universe in which it lives.

The first, and the relative newcomer on the block, is what we know today as science. Ideally, this process involves collecting thousands of bits of information based on observations. From such data, conclusions are drawn and theories are advanced. The shortcoming of this approach is that science cannot deal with things that it can't see—thoughts, motivation, or spirit.

The second major approach starts with set premises and fits one's observations into them. A classic example is Chinese medicine, largely unchanged for the past 4,000 years. Its understanding of the human body is based on three main philosphical concepts. The first is the existence of the Tao (meaning "the way"), which is the path to maintaining harmony and which incorporates the belief of a life force. The second major concept is that this life force, the ch'i, has two polarities, yang and yin, and a balance between them is essential to maintain health. Finally, humans are a microcosm of the macrocosm and, hence, are composed of the five elements—fire, earth, metal, water, and wood. Health and illness are a manifestation of the balance and inner action of these as well.

The shortcoming of this approach is that it often lacks flexibility and has much difficulty in dealing with new pieces of information. For example, two Chinese doctors after watching the autopsy of an English sailor in the nineteenth century, said, "We are overcome by your kindness, but everything we have seen is in complete disagreement with the teaching of our books." After saying this, they left, not wanting to deal with this invasion of their cosmology. More recently, the Chinese have wrestled with the molecular knowledge generated in the West. Vitamin B12 has been pronounced very yang; penicillin, very yin. The point is that there can be nothing beyond yin and yang — everything has to fit into their system.

The roots of Western medicine are found in this latter approach as well. Health and disease 2,500 years ago were viewed as either the gift or the curse of the gods. The god of healing was Aesclepius, son of Apollo. By the time of Alexander the Great, it is estimated that there were between three hundred and four hundred temples dedicated to Aesclepius. Each of these was a "holistic healing" center far beyond anything that exists today. Imagine a large group of springs in the suburbs of Washington, D.C. To this, add a theater with seating capacity of twenty thousand, a stadium 600 feet long with seating for twelve thousand, and all the possible accessories of art and science. You now have an idea of what the temple closest to Athens was like in the third century B.C. Access to these temples was restricted; pilgrims who wished to enter submitted to a process of purification, bathing, and fasting. Specific diets were required. Solemn rituals of prayer and sacrifice accompanied these procedures. This integrated spirit-body approach continued once inside the temple. The priest, also teacher and healer, applied physical measures. An equally important part of this ritual was the incubation sleep. During the dream state, Aesclepius was expected to visit the sick, healing them or prescribing modes of treatment.

Into this setting was born Hippocrates, the son of a priest of Aesclepius.

A great observer, Hippocrates emphasized that diseases were products of natural, not supernatural forces. Supreme was the *vis medicatrix naturae*, the power of nature to heal. For the next 500 years, medicine was a blend of spiritual vision and scientific method. Emotions, personality, and environmental factors were taken into account in diagnosis and treatment of disease.

Times changed with the spread of Christianity in the second and third centuries A.D. Nature was separated as being something different from God; its great forces were ignored or even despised. Man was to be led out of nature toward God above. For the next 1,000 years, the body and its workings were largely ignored. Then times changed again during the Renaissance, when man began again to observe and question the world in which he lived.

During this transition, two important events occurred. The first involved a man named Paracelsus, who incessantly questioned and found fault with the existing assumptions. He so rattled the status quo that flexibility was forced back into the system and, with it, the concept that theories could change over time as new observations were made. The second event was facilitated by René Descartes. At this time, researchers who wanted to investigate the human body found themselves in direct conflict with the Church, which saw such investigation as a desecration of the soul. Descartes pronounced that there was a *res externa* and a *res cogitans*—a body and a soul, each separate from the other. The Church was able to retain ownership of the soul while the scientists could take ownership of the body. This change allowed men like Vesalius to study the body's anatomy in detail and others, like Harvey, to outline its physiology.

The years following these two events were ones of rapidly changing concepts as the body was studied in more and more detail. One culmination of such study was the postulating of the cell theory in 1839 by two German biologists, Schleiden and Schwann. Theirs was the first truly unifying concept in biology, stating that the cell is the fundamental unit of all that is alive. Based on this new concept, other researchers pronounced disease to be a problem that occurs at the level of the cell.

In the last 150 years, this approach has been taken even further—to what is called the molecular theory of disease causation. Disease is now seen as a problem in the balance of molecules inside the cell. Along with this comes the concept that if the right molecules (in the form of medicine) can be added to the body, we should be able to correct the problem.

Application, however, often lags behind understanding and this was very true in medicine. In 1839, when the cell theory was first put forth, the world was in the midst of what was known as the "Age of Heroic Medicine." Disease was believed to be contained in the body's fluids; for healing to occur it was necessary that these fluids be purged. The favorite treatment of the time was bleeding the patient, through the use of leeches or incisions. Also high on the list were herbs that would induce vomiting or profuse sweating. In some cases, huge doses of Calomel were used until the patient started to salivate (now known to be an early sign of mercury poisoning).

The public appears to have figured out the danger of these practices before the profession did. During the 1830s and 1840s, many joined with Jacksonian Democrats to form the very powerful Popular Health Movement. The trend was toward self-responsibility with the slogan, "Every man his own doctor." By the end of the 1840s, this organization had wiped nearly all the licensing laws off the books.

Within a short while the establishment caught on and Oliver Wendell Holmes, the famed Harvard Medical School professor, said "I firmly believe that if the whole *materia medica* as now used could be sunk to the bottom of the sea, it would be all the better for mankind and all the worse for the fishes." In 1876, Edward H. Clarke, one of Holmes' Harvard colleagues, wrote a sober essay reviewing what he regarded as the major scientific accomplishments in medicine during the preceding 50 years. He cited studies of typhoid and typhus fever which proved not only that the patients could recover by themselves without medical intervention, but that they often did better if left alone and not treated with the heavy metals, fomentations, and herbs popular at that time.

With this new understanding, therapy at the end of the nineteenth century became much less ambitious and flamboyant. "Supportive treatment," consisting mainly of common sense, appropriate rest, a sensible diet, and a trust that nature would help correct the situation replaced the reckless methods of the past.

During this transition, numerous alternative therapies sprouted and thrived. In 1900—the year Edgar Cayce gave his first reading—allopathy was far from being the only kid on the block. There were twenty-two homeopathic medical schools in the United States and more than fifteen thousand practitioners of the discipline. The American School of Osteopathy in Kirksville, Missouri, was 8 years old and was attracting new followers daily. The year 1900 also marks establishment of the first college of naturopathy. This discipline returned to the ideas of Hippocrates and his belief in the healing powers of nature. It combined baths, borrowed from European health spas of the day, with herbs, nutrition, psychology, and massage as therapies to aid nature's own processes.

In the midst of this influx of new ideas, Cayce began to give readings. The readings appeared to be in philosophical agreement with the shift in perspective. The Cayce source indicated that all healing was to be found in nature, citing osteopathy and hydrotherapy as the two therapies best for facilitating healing. "For nature is much better *yet* than science!" (no. 759–12)

Then, fairly suddenly, application caught up with understanding and medicine entered the age of the molecule. The power of this change is dramatically illustrated by the story of antibiotics. Penicillin, the first antibiotic, wasn't discovered until 1928. But suddenly with the use of a molecule, diseases that had once plagued mankind were controlled and almost wiped out.

As a result, two dramatic changes occurred in the perspectives of doctors. First, a tremendous sense of optimism took hold. Complicated and devastating diseases like tuberculosis and syphilis were now treatable. The search began for a magic molecule to cure each and every ailment. The second change was that physicians suddenly felt they were scientists. Wishing to distance themselves from the magic of the past, physicians became hardcore materialists. Although the word "physician" stems from the Greek word for "nature," allopathic treatment today depends almost solely on drugs. In fact, the term "medicine" has become synonomous with pharmaceutical products and many people are surprised to learn that there are systems of treatment today which do not use drugs at all. During this time of optimism and materialism, the Cayce physical readings, as well as other alternative therapies, were largely ignored. Faith in science became stronger than faith in nature in American society. A 1964 book sympathetic to homeopathy, osteopathy, and naturopathy, was titled "Fringe Medicine."

Then the winds shifted again. In 1965, noting the increasing popularity of "fringe medicine," medical philosopher René Dubos commented that "its popularity points to the failure of the present biomedical science to satisfy large human needs." As the public scrutinized the profession again, history repeated itself and the prevailing attitudes became similar to those found in the Popular Health Movement during the 1830s and 1840s.

What factors led to this change? First of all, optimism was fading. Despite advances, Americans were living no longer than they had been before. While there were some dramatic successes in the treatment of infectious disease, other diseases like cancer and heart disease took their place. It became evident that the words of Hans Selye—"The more man learns about more ways to combat external causes of death (germs, cold, hunger) the more likely is he to die from his own voluntary suicidal behavior"— were true. Medicine also had become too expensive and too dangerous in light of its diminishing returns. Hospital medicine, with its invasive procedures, began to look more and more like "heroic medicine." Tragedies like the thalidomide babies in the early 1960s made people aware that the molecules they were taking could have terrible side effects. Likewise, the six to twelve thousand deaths per year attributed to drugs and the publicized excesses in surgery speeded the change. In addition, the annual cost of medicine continued to rise at about twice the rate of inflation. From the 3.5 percent of the Gross National Product that health-care costs had been during Cayce's day in the 1920s, health care now consumed more than 10 percent of the GNP.

Allopathy's materialism also was being challenged. While medicine in the last fifty years had attempted to align with the sciences, physics—the "hardest" of sciences—had gone "soft." Physicists announced that the universe could no longer be perceived as an orderly mechanism that was independent of the consciousness of those observing it. Another blow to materialism came from the numerous emerging studies that showed a relationship between the mind and the body.

Despite modern medicine's impressive record of clinical success backed by intellectual prestige, the trappings of modern technology, and vast sums of money, significant numbers of patients have emerged from encounters with medicine during the last 20 years feeling more anger and resentment than gratitude. A 1980 poll showed that the proportion of people who trusted their family doctor dropped below 50 percent for the first time in modern history. In fact, it dropped to less than 40 percent in that single year. As a result, more people today than at any time in the last 50 years are willing to consider alternative forms of therapy.

With this renewed interest, the "fringe medicines" have now become "holistic medicine," although this change has not been a panacea, either. Far from a coherent system of treatment, holistic medicine is an informal collection of attitudes and practices, some of which are bizarre. Two factors seem to hold this movement together: many of its members have a strong anti-allopathic sentiment and all have a strong belief that any healing system needs to consider the mental and spiritual aspects of an individual.

As this brief history hopefully illustrates, interest in the connection between spirit and mind with the physical is not new. Historically, how a society views its spirituality plays a large role in how it approaches healing the body. The substance of present-day holistic medicine has been with us for the last several thousand years; it certainly is not a phenomena that is less than 100 years old.

While the holistic health movement has addressed some vital questions which allopathy has ignored, it has its own significant Achilles' heel. Like Chinese medicine, many of the varied therapies which claim to be part of the holistic health movement begin with certain set premises about the universe and the way it works. As in Chinese medicine, many of these premises incorporate the ideas of a life force and of man as a microcosm of the macrocosm. Also like Chinese medicine, most of these systems have trouble incorporating reality as perceived by science. They largely ignore the principles of causation and repeatability and often can't rectify their conclusions with those based on the observations of science. This has resulted in several unfortunate occurrences. Almost without exception, holistic therapies cannot explain how they work in terms of the physiology and anatomy of the body. As a result, we really don't know which of these therapies work and which don't. Finally, some people have latched onto the holistic health movement as a way to garner power, prestige, and money at the expense of the sick—with very little accountability for their actions.

Let's now return to the question: where do the Edgar Cayce health readings fit into this jumbled mass of varied opinions and approaches to the human body, mind, and spirit? The answer lies directly in the beauty, depth, and consistency of the more than nine thousand physical readings that were given. As in Chinese medicine, there emerges in the readings a coherent philosophy and approach to the body based on spiritual premises about the universe. The readings, however, are also equally at home in the world of the cell and the molecule, agreeing with science that the disease process occurs at this level of our physical bodies. The readings are comfortable in both worlds and can move from a discussion of the kundalini forces to the effects of anger on the body to the balance of electrolytes in the blood. At one moment, they can discuss the physiology of the spirit and, in the next, talk about the workings of the kidneys. The readings, more than 60 years ago, discussed the importance of visualization and relaxation to the healing process—long before the topic was popular. The readings also, however, encourage people to verify the principles that are set forth and give ideas for experimentation to accomplish this.

The information given through Cayce over a 40-year period, in my opinion, contains a remarkable understanding of the anatomy and physiology of the human body. Impressive for their use of technical terms and knowledge, the readings are even more amazing in their presentation of new concepts. Some of these, like the diagnostic possibilities of a single drop of blood, are taken for granted today. Others, like the description of the importance of nerve reflexes in the origin and treatment of asthma, are logical extensions of our current knowledge. However, the readings also contain concepts which are foreign to our current understanding and would be shocking to many physicians. Examples include the role of gold in multiple sclerosis, the importance of the potassium/iodide balance in thyroid disorders, and the place of colonics in the treatment of coronary heart disease. If only half of the ideas in the readings prove true, our perception of the body will be drastically altered and millions of people will be helped.

SELECTED
BIBLIOGRAPHY

Achterberg, Jeanne. *Imagery in Healing: Shamanism and Modern Medicine*. Boston: Shambhala Publications, 1985.

A.R.E. *An Edgar Cayce Home Medicine Guide*. Virginia Beach, Virginia: A.R.E. Press, 1982.

Becker, Robert O., and Gary Selden. *The Body Electric: Electromagnetism and the Foundation of Life*. New York: William Morrow, 1985.

Bennet, Hal Zina. *The Doctor Within*. New York: Clarkson N. Potter, 1981.

Benson, Herbert, and William Proctor. *Beyond the Relaxation Response*. New York: Berkeley, 1985.

Bliss, Shepherd (ed.). *The New Holistic Health Handbook*. Lexington, Massachusetts: Penguin Books, 1985.

Bolduc, Henry Leo. *Self-Hypnosis: Creating Your Own Destiny*. Virginia Bech, Virginia: A.R.E. Press, 1985.

Borysenko, Joan. *Minding the Body, Mending the Mind*. Massachusetts: Addison-Wesley, 1987.

Catalano, Ellen Mohr. *The Chronic Pain Control Workbook: A Step-by-Step Guide for Coping with and Overcoming Your Pain*. Oakland, California: New Harbinger Publications, 1987.

Dossey, Larry. *Space, Time, and Medicine*. Boston: Shambhala Publications, 1982.

Frank, Jerome D. *Persuasion and Healing: A Comparative Study of Psychotherapy*. Baltimore: Johns Hopkins University Press, 1973.

Greenman, Phillip E. *Principles of Manual Medicine*. Baltimore: Williams and Wilkins, 1989.

Hastings, Arthur C., James Fadiman, and James S. Gordon (eds.). *Health for the Whole Person: The Complete Guide to Holistic Medicine*. Boulder, Colorado: Westview Press, 1980.

Karp, Reba Ann. *Edgar Cayce: Encyclopedia of Healing*. New York: Warner Books, 1986.

McGarey, William A. *The Edgar Cayce Remedies*. Toronto: Bantam Books, 1983.

———. *Physician's Reference Notebook*. Virginia Beach, Virginia: A.R.E. Press, 1983.

Puryear, Herbert B., and Mark A. Thurston. *Meditation and the Mind of Man*. Virginia Beach, Virginia: A.R.E. Press, 1975.

Reilly, Harold J., and Ruth Hagy Brod. *The Edgar Cayce Handbook for Health Through Drugless Therapy*. New York: Macmillan, 1975.

Rossi, Ernest L., *The Psychobiology of Mind-Body Healing: New Concepts of Therapeutic Hypnosis*. New York: W. W. Norton, 1986.

Ryan, Regina Sara, and John W. Travis. *The Wellness Workbook*. Berkeley, California: Ten Speed Press, 1981.

Siegel, Bernie S. *Love, Medicine, and Miracles*. New York: Harper & Row, 1986.

Thrash, Agatha, and Calvin Thrash. *Home Remedies: Hydrotherapy, Massage, Charcoal, and Other Simple Treatments*. Searle, Alabama: Thrash Publications, 1981.

Weil, Andrew. *Health and Healing: Understanding Conventional and Alternative Medicine*. Boston: Houghton Mifflin, 1983.

INDEX

ABOUT THE
AUTHOR

Eric A. Mein, M.D., has a special interest in the interrelationship of spirit, mind, and body in both health and disease. In preparation for this book, Dr. Mein spent a year as a visiting scholar at the Edgar Cayce Foundation researching the Cayce readings' perspective on this relationship.

To pursue his findings, Dr. Mein has founded Meridian Institute (P.O. Box 1479, Virginia Beach, VA 23451). The goal of this organization is to help expand the meeting ground between science and spirit by sponsoring clinical and basic science research, which examines concepts about the body that are compatible with the premise that we are spiritual beings and approach the healing process from that perspective.

Dr. Mein lives in Seattle, Washington, with his wife Cathy and their two children, Rachael and Christopher.

EDGAR CAYCE'S
WISDOM FOR THE NEW AGE

More information from the Edgar Cayce readings is available to you on hundreds of topics from astrology and arthritis to universal laws and world affairs, because Cayce's friends established an organization, the Association for Research and Enlightenment (A.R.E.), to facilitate his readings and make the information available for research.

Today over seventy-five thousand members of the A.R.E. receive the bimonthly magazine *Venture Inward*, which contains articles on dream interpretation, past lives, health and diet tips, psychic archaeology, and psi research, as well as book reviews and interviews with leaders and authors in the metaphysical field. Members also receive extracts of medical and nonmedical readings and may do their own research in all of the over fourteen thousand readings that Edgar Cayce gave during his lifetime.

To receive more information about the association that continues to research and make available information on subjects in the Edgar Cayce readings, please write A.R.E., Dept. M13, P.O. Box 595, Virginia Beach, VA 23451, or call (804) 428-3588. The A.R.E. will be happy to send you a packet of materials describing its current activities.